NATURAL
Alternatives
to Antibiotics

Dr. John McKenna

AVERY PUBLISHING GROUP

Garden City Park • New York

The therapeutic procedures in this book are based on the training, experiences, and research of the author. Because each person and situation are unique, the author and publisher urge the reader to check with a qualified health professional before using any procedure where there is any question to appropriateness.

The publisher does not advocate the use of any particular health program, but believes the information presented in this book should be available to the public.

Because there is always some risk involved, the author and publisher are not responsible for any adverse effects or consequences resulting from the use of any of the suggestions or preparations in this book. Please do not use the book if you are unwilling to assume the risk. Feel free to consult with a physician or other qualified health professional. It is a sign of wisdom, not cowardice, to seek a second or third opinion.

Cover designers: Doug Brooks
    and William Gonzalez
Cover photo: Photodisc
In-house editor: Dara Stewart
Typesetter: Helen Contoudis

Avery Publishing Group
120 Old Broadway
Garden City Park, NY 11040
1-800-548-5757
www.averypublishing.com

Library of Congress Cataloging-in-Publication Data

McKenna, John, Dr.
    Natural alternatives to antibiotics : using nature's pharmacy to help fight infections / John McKenna.
    Rev. ed. of: Alternatives to antibiotics. Dublin : Gill & Macmillan, 1996.
    p. cm.
    Includes bibliographical references and index.
    ISBN 0-89529-839-2
    1. Communicable diseases—Alternative treatment. 2. Drug resistance in microorganisms. 3. Naturopathy. 4. Homeopathy. 5. Herbs—Therapeutic use. 6. Dietary supplements. I. McKenna, John, Dr. Alternatives to antibiotics. II. Title.
RC112.M39 1998   98-26253
616.9'046—dc21   CIP

Printed in the United States of America

10 9 8 7 6 5 4

CONTENTS

ACKNOWLEDGMENTS

I would like to thank my good friend David Niket Ring for helping to guide me through a very difficult period in my life. His wisdom has enabled me to see the importance of making certain changes, including writing this book and expressing what I feel more publicly.

I would also like to thank another friend, Angela Leahy, for her constant encouragement and belief in me and for helping me with many aspects of the preparation of the original draft.

My practice nurse, Joan Deegan, also deserves thanks for helping me to keep the practice going while I was working such long hours on this book. Her care, compassion, understanding, and common sense made it a pleasure to work with her.

Thanks also go to Siobhán for her pleasant approach, for covering for Joan, and for making it possible for me to get on with my research. My thanks to John Doyle for many things, especially for proofreading the final script.

I did not realize the importance of a good editor until I worked with both Roberta Reeners and Karin Whooley. In spite of having little medical knowledge, they helped me to get my message across in a simple and effective way. My apologies to Aisling Collins for not being able to use her evocative illustrations this time.

Thanks to Wendy MacDonnell and to Hansen Laboratories for their help with research information; to Merck, Sharp, and Dohme for the use of *Antibiotics in Historical Perspective*, and to Schaper and Brümmer for help with research and for slides of certain herbs.

I am grateful to all my patients for their support over the past five years. It is because of them that this book came about. Without their help, a simpler and gentler form of medicine would not be possible. Particular thanks to those who agreed to let me use their case histories.

My greatest debt of gratitude is to my family, who has borne the pain of long periods of separation with great strength.

FOREWORD

It was after a talk in Dublin that I first had the pleasure of meeting Dr. John McKenna. During our conversation, John told me he was writing this book—its publication could not have come at a more important time. It is a long-awaited and necessary book, which addresses many issues and answers many questions.

Nowadays, people have a better understanding of the side effects related to the long-term use of antibiotics. Back in 1958, when I received my degree in pharmacy, it was not a subject for public concern. The issue was on my mind even then, however. At that particular time, there was an explosion in the use of antibiotics, tranquilizers, and sleeping tablets. Since then, development of these drugs has continued unabated, and today, when I look at the numerous patients I treat in my seven British clinics, I understand even better what I saw happening in the late fifties.

This book describes the many alternatives available. Echinacea, for example, was recently shown to be one of the best natural antibiotics in a study at the University of München in Germany. My own partner, Dr. Alfred Vogel, now 95 years old and still skiing, has been promoting echinacea for more than forty years, and I am delighted that he can now see a scientific report validating its great benefits. This report proves that there *are* natural ways to support and boost the defenses of the human body.

Some time ago, I was asked to speak to a group of doctors and medical students in Germany. While talking about the immune system, I briefly mentioned a product called Echinaforce, the fresh herb extract from *Echinacea purpurea*. The doctors in question were very interested in the methods I have been using during the past thirty-five years to ease human suffering. I was especially pleased when, at the end of my lecture, one doctor stood up to endorse what I had said about echinacea. Apparently, while traveling in Brazil, she had acquired a nasty throat infection. As there was no pharmacy nearby, she was unable to obtain antibiotics, so she bought a bottle of Echinaforce in a simple health-food store instead. As she believed it could not do the job, she took twice the recommended dosage and found, to her surprise, that her sore throat had eased considerably by evening. Since then, she has prescribed echinacea to many of her patients, with great success.

This clearly and concisely written book is a timely reminder of the great possibilities that nature has to offer. Nature is balanced and will always have the power to heal. The many subjects that Dr. John McKenna discusses in this book open the way to a greater recognition and understanding of natural remedies. After all, we are born in nature and have to obey the laws of nature if we want to stay healthy and fit. I am happy to see more and more people throughout the world becoming aware of the natural options available to them, instead of using and abusing synthetic antibiotics.

I am sure that the readers of this book will be impressed and rewarded by the tremendous research and knowledge that has gone into its publication.

Jan de Vries, D.Ho.Med.,
D.O.M.R.O., N.D.M.R.N., D.Ac., M.B.Ac.A.

PREFACE

Antibiotics are drugs that are used to treat infections. A whole range of antibiotics have been produced since the 1940s, when they were first developed. They are now among the most commonly prescribed drugs in the world.

Antibiotics act by killing or controlling the growth of the germ that is causing a disease. They are very effective in combating infections caused by bacteria, like strep throat (a streptococcal infection), for example. They are absolutely *useless* in treating infections caused by viruses, such as influenza or the common cold.

The real value of antibiotics is in sharp decline today because they have been abused worldwide. Reports in recent years show an ever-increasing problem of resistance to antibiotics emerging in different parts of the world. As people become more aware of this and of the side effects of antibiotics, they are demanding alternatives. This book describes those alternatives in detail. Natural medicines, especially herbal and homeopathic medicines, are coming back in vogue and are regaining their rightful place in providing a balanced way of treating infection. People are becoming much more conscious of the foods they eat and are aware of the need for food supplements, especially vitamins and minerals. All of these topics, as well as case histories to illustrate the way in which specific infections can be treated by natural means, make this book a valuable asset to any household. It is especially important for the parents of children who suffer from recurrent infections.

Because this book is aimed at the general public, it has been kept as simple as possible, with a minimum of scientific or medical jargon. It is designed to show that it is possible to treat infections without antibiotics, but it does not deny the fact that antibiotics may sometimes be needed. This, however, is the exception rather than the rule. This book is not suggesting that you stay away from your doctor. Rather, you should visit your doctor and encourage your doctor to use natural methods whenever possible.

When choosing a doctor, try to find one who is open to the use of natural methods as well as conventional medicine. Since many of the medicines discussed in this book will be available only by prescription, it is best to go to practitioners who can prescribe them.

The aim of this book is to bring some common sense back into clinical medicine and to support a gentler way of healing people. The first part of the book deals with the history and development of antibiotics, their conventional usage, and the much publicized issue of antibiotic resistance. Later, I deal with some of the common infections in children. The greater part of the book, however, looks at alternative methods of treating infections, from herbal medicine to homeopathy to nutritional medicine.

The case histories have been selected from my own practice for the purpose of illustrating my particular point of view. All the names have been changed to protect the confidentiality of the patients concerned. I could include many cases of a more dramatic nature, such as the one in the Introduction. However, I have chosen to keep the case histories simple so that they do not overshadow my purpose in writing, which is to illustrate the value of the different forms of alternative medicine in treating infections.

INTRODUCTION

Here are the clinical records of a (then) 14-year-old boy. He was born in January of 1980.

Date	Prescription	Type of Drug
09/1980	Keflex (cephalexin)	Antibiotic
01/1981	Septra (trimethoprim and sulfamethoxazole)	Antibiotic
05/1981	Chlorpheniramine maleate	Antihistamine
07/1981	Thenoxymetyll penicillin	Antibiotic
12/1981	Bactrim (trimethoprim and sulfamethoxazole)	Antibiotic
01/1982	Bactrim (trimethoprim and sulfamethoxazole)	Antibiotic
03/1982	Keflex (cephalexin)	Antibiotic
05/1982	Amoxil (amoxicillin)	Antibiotic
09/1982	Oxacillin	Antibiotic
04/1983	Keflex (cephalexin)	Antibiotic
04/1983	Amoxil (amoxicillin)	Antibiotic
06/1983	EryPed (erythromycin ethylsuccinate)	Antibiotic

Date	Prescription	Type of Drug
08/1983	Amoxil (amoxicillin)	Antibiotic
08/1983	Hydrocortisone cream	Steroid
09/1983	EryPed (erythromycin ethylsuccinate)	Antibiotic
09/1983	Metoclopramide	Anti-nausea drug
10/1983	Keflex (cephalexin)	Antibiotic
11/1983	Hydrocortisone cream	Steroid
12/1983	Vallergan syrup*	Antihistamine
01/1984	Keflex (cephalexin)	Antibiotic
04/1984	Keflex (cephalexin)	Antibiotic
06/1984	Keflex (cephalexin)	Antibiotic
06/1984	Alupent (metaproterenol sulfate)	Bronchodilator (dilates airways in asthmatics)
07/1984	Keflex (cephalexin)	Antibiotic
09/1984	EryPed (erythromycin ethylsuccinate)	Antibiotic
10/1984	Diprosone cream*	Potent steroid
11/1984	Vallergan*	Antihistamine
12/1984	Ceporex (cephalexin)	Antibiotic
01/1985	Ceporex (cephalexin)	Antibiotic
01/1985	Diprosone cream	Potent steroid
02/1985	Amoxil (amoxicillin)	Antibiotic
06/1985	Amoxil (amoxicillin)	Antibiotic
07/1985	Triludan syrup*	Antihistamine
09/1985	Keflex (cephalexin)	Antibiotic
09/1985	Ventolin (albuterol)	Bronchodilator
10/1985	Distaclor*	Antibiotic
10/1985	Ventolin (albuterol)	Bronchodilator
11/1985	Amoxil (amoxicillin)	Antibiotic
11/1985	Ventolin (albuterol)	Bronchodilator

Date	Prescription	Type of Drug
12/1985	Amoxil (amoxicillin)	Antibiotic
01/1986	Hydrocortisone cream	Steroid
01/1986	Fucidin cream (fucidic acid)	Antibiotic
01/1986	Ceporex (cephalexin)	Antibiotic
02/1986	Keflex (cephalexin)	Antibiotic
02/1986	Ventolin (albuterol)	Bronchodilator
03/1986	Ventolin (albuterol)	Bronchodilator
04/1986	Ventolin (albuterol)	Bronchodilator
04/1986	EryPed (erythromycin ethylsuccinate)	Antibiotic

* United Kingdom brand name.

This child was given his first antibiotic when he was 9 months old. Before he had reached his seventh birthday, he had received no less than *thirty* courses of antibiotics. He was diagnosed as being asthmatic in September of 1985.

These antibiotics were prescribed for sore throats, coughs, bronchitis, and as a "precaution" when the child had a wheezy chest. The steroids were prescribed for allergic rashes—which may well have been caused by the antibiotics!

This senseless use of antibiotics, one course after the next, after the next, after the next, must be condemned. Remember, this is a young child who was being given these drugs. It could have been *your* child, and, as this book will show you, these drugs are far from harmless.

This, however, is not the worst case I have encountered. I am alarmed by this. As patients, parents, or interested readers, you are probably alarmed too. *You* are the ones who have alerted me to this problem and who have asked me for a better method of treatment.

Early in 1994, I gave a series of talks entitled "How to Treat Infections Without Antibiotics." These talks attracted considerable attention, so much so that it became apparent to me that people wanted to know a lot more about this subject. It was at these talks that I was encouraged to put my approach on paper—hence this book.

I do not quote the above case history to criticize the medical profession, the child's doctor, or his parents. Nor do I want to highlight the inherent difficulty in trying to treat infections with antibiotics alone. Believe me, there are safe, effective alternatives available. Open your mind and read the research. Above all, try the alternatives. It is only by trying alternatives that you will learn for yourself, as I have had to. I am privileged to have had wonderful patients who have continuously supported me in my work through their understanding, their belief, and their patience. They have taught me much, especially about myself, and I thank them.

This boy's case history suggests that a more broad-minded approach to the causes of recurrent infections is needed. Treating the symptoms is often fruitless and does damage to everyone concerned. Locating the underlying causes is the only way to treat such a child. This child's case also reflects the need for a less scientific, more humane, caring, and compassionate approach to medicine—put another way, an approach using more of the heart and less of the head. The head without the heart results in a form of medicine that is cold and unsympathetic to human suffering. It lacks wisdom and understanding of the consequences of treating people in this way. The global problem of resistance to antibiotics would not have arisen if we had placed more emphasis on this wisdom and understanding, and less on accepted scientific knowledge. Knowledge, when guided by the wisdom handed down to us from past generations, will guarantee a future. But to accept and understand this wisdom, you must open your heart.

Many doctors know very little about alternative medicine, yet they are quick to say it does not work. For example, while working at the Royal Victoria Hospital in Belfast, Ireland, I heard a consultant surgeon from Scotland condemn acupuncture as nonsense and quackery. This is sad to hear. The research done to date clearly shows that acupuncture works.

Conventional medicine is very much disease-oriented, almost to the point of viewing the disease as separate from the patient. As a consequence of this, infections are approached from a curative point of view; drugs that kill the bacterium or fungus are used to cure the disease. So if two patients have the same infection, such as a streptococcal sore throat, they will receive the same treatment.

This curative, or antimicrobial, approach to treating an infection seldom looks at the reasons why the infection has arisen in the first place. Finding these reasons is of vital importance when it comes to prevention. The underlying reasons why infections occur, and particularly why they recur, may be related to a weakened immune system in one patient, to poor nutrition in another, and to emotional stress or trauma in yet another. The conventional approach uses an antibiotic to treat not just the initial infection, but all infections thereafter as well. If one antibiotic does not work, others are tried.

Despite the side effects associated with these drugs, courses of antibiotics are readily and frequently prescribed. This illustrates a fundamental weakness in medical training, with doctors being taught only this particular approach to treating infections. Many general practitioners are caught in this trap. Their training has focused on the use of drugs, but many of them feel increasingly uncomfortable with the drug-based approach and are looking for alternatives.

Practitioners of alternative medicine seek to treat not only the particular infection that a patient exhibits, but also the patient. Alternative medicine provides both doctor and patient with a more personalized approach to treatment than conventional medicine.

Alternative medicine is more patient-oriented and views the patient in much broader terms than does conventional medicine. It takes account of the fact that you are not just a physical body. It recognizes the fact that you have a mind, or mental body, with a particular set of thought patterns that affects the way you view everything around you. It recognizes that you have an emotional body that has a strong interaction with your physical body; anger raises your blood pressure significantly, for example. Alternative medicine also recognizes that you have a soul, or spiritual body, which is the very core of your being. Any form of medicine that recognizes and treats these different levels of being facilitates a better understanding of the origins of many illnesses and of ourselves. A very good example of interaction between mind and body is discussed in Chapter 10, which deals with stress.

Since it is very broad in its approach, alternative medicine is able to be both curative and preventative. This approach could even be regarded as being more preventative than curative because it looks beyond the patient's symptoms and attempts to locate the underlying causes of an infection. As a result, it is often better able to prevent the recurrence of an illness. Treatment with natural immune-enhancing medicines, certain homeopathic medicines, and vitamin/mineral supplements helps to ensure that an illness does not recur.

The natural approach to medical treatment educates patients and gives them more control over their own health. It also breaks the vicious cycle of dependence on one antibiotic after another. Because alternative medicines are natural, they are also, for the most part, free of side effects.

Although these two approaches are quite different, they share the same goal, helping you, the patient. If both conventional and alternative practitioners can keep the patient in the foreground and their own vested interests in the background, we will all benefit. Conventional doctors can learn from alternative practitioners and the latter can benefit from the medical research, the laboratory investigations, and the access to emergency backup services of conventional medicine.

Open-mindedness and a willingness to respect another approach to healing is the way forward. I believe that neither approach is inherently wrong. Both have much to offer a patient and each other. I believe that the future in medicine lies in incorporating both forms of medicine into a system of healing in which the intuitive ability of a healer is developed alongside the healer's scientific skills. The art of healing must combine with the science of medicine if we are to prevent disease whenever possible, and to wisely treat those problems that do occur.

It is important that you and I speak from the heart and say what we feel is right, even in the face of aggressive contradiction. It is also important to convert your local doctor and continually insist on safer medicine. The same message heard repeatedly and from different sources eventually has an impact. If you say nothing, medicine will not change. Then you, or your child, may be the recipient of the kind of treatment described earlier. It is time for you to choose.

A safer form of medicine and a gentler approach to patients are what I stand for. If this is what you stand for, then say so. By doing this, you encourage change. I believe in people; the more information and power people have, the more common sense will prevail. The purpose of this book is to inform people about the medical issues confronting us today. I hope you will both enjoy it and learn more by reading it.

CHAPTER 1

THE HISTORY OF ANTIBIOTICS

The Gold Rush

Antibiotics, in one form or another, have been in use for centuries. Prehistoric man may not have realized why or how the wide variety of organic and inorganic substances he used worked. The important thing was that these substances did, indeed, work. Before the advent of commercial antibiotics, a common-sense approach to infection was obviously being used: do little to treat the infection initially, allow the body to fight it naturally, and in so doing, build up one's natural resistance to it. Only when the body clearly was not winning the battle was intervening action taken.

In general, people depended on herbal medicines and folk cures. Ireland had a strong tradition of herbal medicine, with a doctor or herbalist ready to help in the treatment of infections. As in many other cultures, the knowledge of growing and using herbal medicines was handed down from generation to generation. Doctors depended, to a great extent, on natural substances such as iron, mercury, and antimony.

It was not until the nineteenth century that scientists began to closely examine various curative substances in order to understand exactly how and why they were effective. In the course of this study, scientists discovered that there were beneficial bacteria. They began to experiment, isolating the "good" bacteria and encouraging their growth in the laboratory. These bacterial agents were then tested for their ability to treat disease. This pattern of research and clinical trials continued into the twentieth century (and, in fact, continues today), leading to the production of the first antibiotic drugs.

This chapter outlines the history of antibiotics, from ancient times to the present.

FROM ANCIENT TIMES TO THE NINETEENTH CENTURY

The earliest evidence of humans using plants or other natural substances for therapeutic purposes, comes from the Neanderthals, who lived over 50,000 years ago. In northern Iraq, archaeologists uncovered evidence of human remains that had been buried with a range of herbs, some of which are now known to be antibacterial—that is, used to kill bacteria or to prevent them from multiplying. Many of these herbs are still used by the inhabitants of this region today. And in other regions, many other antibacterial substances—both organic and inorganic—have been used over time.

Honey

The first prescription for treating infections may well have come from the Egyptians around 1550 BC. Written as "mrht," "byt," and "ftt," it was a mixture of lard, honey, and lint, and was used as an ointment for dressing wounds.

We know that honey is antibacterial—it kills bacterial cells by drawing water out of them. In addition, the enzyme inhibine, which is found in honey, converts glucose and oxygen into hydrogen peroxide, a well-known disinfectant.

At the present time, I have a patient who has surface wounds on the ankles, wrists, and elbows. These wounds are very resistant to treatment with antibiotics, but honey heals them with little difficulty. I have found that honey is also excellent for treating infected varicose ulcers.

Tincta in melle linamenta was a regular prescription in Roman times. It is essentially the same ointment that the Egyptians used, with honey as the active ingredient. The Greeks also used honey in wound dressings, often combining it with copper oxide. More recently, during World War II, an ointment of honey and lard was used in Shanghai to treat wounds and skin infections, and with very good results.

Antibacterial Botanicals

Honey was not the only antibacterial substance used by the Egyptians. Fragrant resins, such as frankincense and myrrh, were used to preserve human remains. Onions, which also have antibacterial properties, have often been found in the body cavities of mummies.

The anti-infective properties of onions and garlic were confirmed by researchers in the 1940s. A substance called allicin was isolated in these plants and was shown to be highly effective in killing bacteria.

Another plant, the radish, is also thought to have been used therapeutically by the Egyptians. The anti-infective property of this plant was confirmed with the isolation of raphanin, a substance that has significant antibacterial activity against a broad range of infections.

Molds

The work of Alexander Fleming in the 1920s showed that molds, such as *Penicillium spp.*, can produce antibacterial chemicals. But the use of molds dates back to the ancient Egyptians, and perhaps even earlier. An Egyptian physician, quoted in the Ebers Papyrus around 1550 BC, stated that if a "wound rots . . . then bind on it spoiled barley bread." Indeed, the Egyptians used all kinds of molds to treat surface infections. The ancient Chinese also used molds to treat boils, carbuncles, and other skin infections.

Wine and Vinegar

Wine and vinegar have been popular treatments for infected wounds since the time of Hippocrates. Vinegar is an acid and a powerful antiseptic—a substance that kills the germs that cause disease. The antibacterial properties of wine cannot be fully attributed to its alcohol content, as this is very low. Recent chemical analysis of wine has brought to light the presence of an antibacterial substance called malvoside. It is this substance that is now thought to give wine its antibacterial properties.

Copper

Inorganic substances have also been used to treat infections throughout the ages. Copper was widely used by the Egyptians, Greeks, and Romans, often in combination with honey. Modern scientific tests have proven that copper is indeed antibacterial. For example, a skin infection known as impetigo, which is caused by the *Staphylococcus aureus* bacteria, is currently being treated in France with Eau Dalibour, a combination of zinc and copper. This prescription dates from the time of Jacques Dalibour, surgeon general of the army of Louis XIV, but it may well have been part of French folk medicine long before this.

Antibiotics in Other Parts of Ancient Africa

In his book *The Antibiotic Paradox*, Dr. Stuart Levy mentions the discovery in Africa of 1,000-year-old mummies on which traces of tetracycline (a modern antibiotic) were found. Some of the grains used also contained traces of tetracycline, and microorganisms producing this antibiotic were found in soil samples taken from the area. Had these people discovered tetracycline and used it over the centuries? If so, why was bacterial resistance not a problem for them—or was it?

THE NINETEENTH AND
EARLY TWENTIETH CENTURIES

The nineteenth and early twentieth centuries saw the discovery and development of many new antibiotics. Most were discovered as doctors and scientists worked to isolate and develop "good" bacteria that could be used in the treatment of infectious diseases. Many different antibiotic substances were discovered and developed. This section discusses the processes involved in finding them. Each group of antibiotics is discussed at length as well.

Homeopathy

Homeopathy is the use of minute amounts of substances that would normally cause illness in a healthy person to accelerate the disease process in a sick person in order to treat the illness. In Germany, there is a tradition of homeopathic medicine. Many doctors were trained in the art of homeopathy, and there were a number of lay homeopaths as well.

From the mid-1800s until the turn of the century, homeopathic medicine was extremely popular in Europe and North America. However, as pharmaceutical companies began to rise, conventional medicine began to take a stronghold on medical care. Much of the infrastructure associated with conventional medicine—hospitals, medical schools, research and diagnostic facilities, X-ray machines, etc.—were sponsored by pharmaceutical companies, so as pharmaceutical companies began to dominate the medical field, so, too, did conventional medicine. In the early 1900s, the American Medical Association (AMA) secured a strong political lobby to close many homeopathic colleges and hospitals. By 1920, the number of these American hospitals had dropped to a mere seven.

The AMA had found a powerful ally in pharmaceutical companies, which may explain the AMA's considerable political clout. It may also explain why most medical research is sponsored by pharmaceutical companies and why medical students are taught pharmacology (the use of drugs) as the primary means of treating patients.

Good Bacteria

During the nineteenth century, various experiments were done in an attempt to find a magic, powerful antibacterial substance that would rid humankind of the scourge of infection. In 1877, experiments in Paris demonstrated the benefits of using harmless, "good" bacteria to treat pathogenic or harmful bacteria. These experiments did indeed prove that harmless bacteria could be used to compete with pathogens (harmful bacteria), although they did not kill the pathogens.

Also in Paris, Louis Pasteur described the beneficial effects of injecting animals with harmless soil bacteria to combat anthrax. Many other experiments on anthrax and cholera confirmed these findings and proved that harmless bacteria can inhibit the growth of disease-causing bacteria. In Chapter 8, you will read about the beneficial effects of eating "live" yogurt, which contains "good" bacteria. These "good" bacteria assist the body by producing certain vitamins, while at the same time protecting the body from the growth of harmful, disease-causing bacteria.

Pyocyanase

In Germany in 1888, an antibacterial substance called pyocyanase was isolated. Animal trials of this substance showed it to be very effective. In fact, the results were so exciting that trials were undertaken in humans suffering from a variety of infections. However, the results of the human trials were very disappointing—pyocyanase was found to be too toxic. Consequently, all research on this substance halted.

Salvarsan

In 1910, a more promising agent called salvarsan, which was

actually a dye, was shown to be effective in the treatment of syphilis, a common sexually transmitted disease at the time. Again, toxicity in humans was a major barrier to its development and widespread use.

The problem of toxicity and the failure to find other antimicrobial agents were the two factors hindering the progress of researchers. Enthusiasm began to wane in the search for the "magic bullet" that would rid humanity of infectious diseases, many of which were major causes of death at that time.

The Penicillin Era

The tide began to change when Alexander Fleming discovered penicillin. After distinguishing himself in his medical studies, Dr. Fleming started research work in pathology in 1908. His early work led to the isolation of lysozyme, an enzyme in human tears and nasal mucus. This enzyme proved to be mildly antibacterial, but it was not very effective against most human infections.

In 1928, while attempting to grow the bacteria *Staphylococcus spp.* on an agar plate (a dish used for preparing bacterial cultures), Fleming noticed that the growth of this bacterium was inhibited by a mold that had accidentally contaminated the plate. He decided to identify the mold, which was eventually called *Penicillium notatum*. Fleming was excited by this discovery. He cultured the mold in a special broth and injected the broth into some of his patients, who had various infectious diseases. The results were encouraging, and the broth proved to be nontoxic. Unfortunately, though, Fleming had not made enough of this broth, making his experiment rather limited. When he presented a paper on his findings in 1929, his colleagues in the medical profession were not particularly impressed or interested.

It took two other gifted researchers—Doctors Florey and Chain, working at Oxford University in the late 1930s and early 1940s—to realize the importance of Dr. Fleming's findings. It was their pioneering work that brought penicillin into clinical use. Florey, an Australian doctor, had gone to Oxford on a scholarship to study pathology. Chain was a German chemist who had fled from the Nazis in the 1930s and had come to rest in England.

Florey was eager to form a group of researchers who were interested in finding effective antibacterial substances. He was the microbiologist and clinician, while Chain was the chemist capable of isolating, purifying, and studying the properties of such substances. Their research team was made up of twenty of the best scientists in Britain at that time. They focused their attention on the work of Alexander Fleming and worked at purifying penicillin and testing its effectiveness.

In one laboratory experiment, the team injected fifty mice with a lethal dose of the *Streptococci spp.* bacteria. Twenty-five of these animals received frequent injections of penicillin. The control group (the other twenty-five mice) was not injected with penicillin. After ten days, twenty-four of the twenty-five penicillin-treated mice had survived. All mice in the control group were dead. These startling results were reported in the well-known medical journal *The Lancet* on August 24, 1940.

In 1941, the Oxford group conducted their first clinical trial of penicillin. Their patient was a 43-year-old policeman who was suffering from septicemia (blood poisoning). The man was dying, so Florey and Chain decided to try the seemingly drastic measure of injecting penicillin intramuscularly every three hours for five days. Within twenty-four hours, there was a marked improvement in the man's condition. By the fourth day, his fever was gone and he was eating again. However, after the fifth day, the supply of penicillin ran out and the patient's condition started to deteriorate again. He eventually died. Despite his death, it was clear to all that penicillin was extremely effective at fighting infection.

The Oxford group's next challenge was finding a way to

produce penicillin in large, economical quantities. All efforts to get industrial support for their research in Britain were fruitless, so in the summer of 1941, they went to the United States. Here they succeeded in getting a number of pharmaceutical companies involved in the industrial production of penicillin, including Merck, Squibb, Pfizer, Abbott, Winthrop, and Commercial Solvents. It was these American pharmaceutical companies that made penicillin a therapeutic reality.

Subsequent clinical trials produced spectacular results. Penicillin demonstrated remarkable effectiveness against a range of infections, including pneumonia, septicemia, scarlet fever, strep throat, diphtheria, gonorrhea, and rheumatic fever. There was a general belief that it could help treat any disease—a myth that still exists today. Tremendous publicity surrounded this new "miracle drug," and in 1945, Fleming, Florey, and Chain were jointly awarded the Nobel Prize in Physiology and Medicine.

Penicillin was later produced in oral form and was added to many products, including salves, throat lozenges, nasal ointments, and cosmetic creams. Prior to 1955, its sale was not controlled, so anyone could buy it over the counter without a prescription. This excessive and uncontrolled use led to the overgrowth of resistant bacteria, and the damage had been done. Resistance had become a major problem, and epidemics of staphylococcal-resistant infections began to emerge in hospitals.

Sulfonamides

In 1935, a German researcher showed that a dye called Prontosil Red cured mice that were infected with *Streptococcus spp.* (the bacteria that causes strep throat). Prontosil Red was the precursor of a group of antibiotic-like drugs called sulfonamides, or sulfa drugs. These drugs are still in use today. Septra, for example, which contains sulfamethoxazole, is used to treat respiratory and urinary tract infections.

Streptomycin

Microbiologists have long known that soil contains very few bacteria that are capable of causing infections in humans. The study of soil bacteria and the reasons why they are not more capable of causing disease was the lifelong work of Selman Waksman, a research scientist at Rutgers University in New Jersey.

In 1939, Merck and Company provided Waksman with financial assistance to mount a search for antibiotics in soil microorganisms. In 1943, this search culminated in the isolation of streptomycin, the first antibiotic to offer hope to patients with tuberculosis (TB). This antibiotic is still used today in the treatment of TB..

After clinical use in tuberculosis patients, it was soon realized that streptomycin caused side effects not seen with penicillin, including kidney damage and deafness. However, the main problem encountered in the use of streptomycin, and the one that restricted its effectiveness, was resistance. The speed at which bacteria were able to develop resistance to the drug was a surprise to Waksman and his coworkers. Because of this, they were prompted to search for other antibiotics. This search resulted in the development of neomycin, a drug commonly used in antibacterial ointments today.

Chloramphenicol

In 1947, the antibiotic chloramphenicol was used in a clinical trial to treat an epidemic of typhus in Bolivia. Its success in curbing the epidemic led to its use on the other side of the world—treating scrub typhus in Malaysia.

In the Bolivian epidemic, all twenty-two patients who received chloramphenicol recovered. Of the fifty patients for whom the antibiotic was unavailable, fourteen died. The trial in Bolivia is not the only South American link with this antibiotic. Chloramphenicol was first isolated from a soil sample in Caracas, Venezuela, a discovery that was important in two ways. First, it identified a new antibiotic substance; second, as the clinical trial showed, chloramphenicol could cure previously untreatable diseases, such as typhus. Later, this same antibiotic showed remarkable results in the treatment of typhoid fever. At last scientists were finding effective substances that could treat serious infections.

The euphoria surrounding the discovery of chloramphenicol was dampened somewhat when it was shown to cause serious side effects. By 1950, many investigators had become alarmed by the mounting evidence linking it with serious blood disorders, including anemia and leukemia.

Today, the use of chloramphenicol is limited in developed countries, where more expensive but safer drugs are available. In developing countries, however, it is still widely used because it is so inexpensive to produce. It is used mainly to treat typhus, typhoid fever, meningitis, and brucellosis, but it can also be used for other infections. You may have used it yourself—in ear drops or eye drops.

The Cephalosporins

In the mid-1940s, Giuseppe Brotzu, rector of the University of Cagliari in Sardinia, isolated an antibiotic-like substance from a mold. He conducted clinical trials with the substance (albeit in an impure form) and achieved very good results, particularly in the treatment of staphylococcal infections and in typhoid fever.

Brotzu published his results in 1948, and his work came to the attention of Florey's research group in Oxford. When they obtained samples of the fungus, they were able to isolate and purify several penicillin-like antibiotics. These were called cephalosporins. The cephalosporins are very effective in treating a wide range of bacterial infections. They destroy bacteria in a manner similar to penicillin and are valuable alternatives, especially where resistance to penicillin is a problem. The added advantage is that they have very low toxicity, although allergic reactions develop in about 5 percent of patients.

Modifications of the basic cephalosporin chemical structure led to the development of a whole range of these antibiotics for clinical use. Research into the development of new cephalosporins continues today.

The Tetracyclines

In 1947, chlortetracycline was isolated from a Missouri River mud sample by Benjamin M. Duggar. Chlortetracycline was the first tetracycline, but Duggar's discovery has led to the isolation and subsequent development of a large number of very powerful antibiotics, which now rank second only to the penicillins in their use worldwide.

Because they are active against a broad range of bacteria and are relatively inexpensive to produce, the tetracyclines quickly gained favor and are now used to treat a long list of infections.

The extensive research done on the tetracyclines has shown them to be effective. However, they are also known to cause a number of toxic side effects. The tetracyclines form calcium complexes in growing bone, which may lead to lifelong discoloration and enamel defects in teeth, as well as reduced bone growth. Tetracyclines also cross the placenta and have a greater toxicity in the fetus. As a result of these side effects, they are prohibited in the treatment of infections in pregnant women and in children below the age of seven, as they may inhibit small children's growth.

Other toxic effects include overgrowth of the *Candida spp.* and *Staphylococcus spp.* bacteria in the bowel, leading to chronic infections with these organisms. Liver and kidney damage may also occur in some patients, as may allergic reactions such as hives, skin rash, asthma, and contact dermatitis.

Because the tetracycline antibiotics form complexes with

calcium, magnesium, and iron, they should not be taken with dairy products or any mineral and vitamin supplements containing calcium, magnesium, or iron.

Table 1.1 summarizes the discovery and development of the first and second generations of antibiotics during the 1940s and 1960s.

Table 1.1 Antibiotics Discovered and Developed in the 1940s and 1960s

First generation of antibiotics	
1942	Penicillin developed
1943	Streptomycin discovered
1945	Cephalosporins discovered
1947	Chloramphenicol discovered
1947	Chlortetracycline discovered
Second generation of antibiotics	
1960	Methicillin developed
1961	Ampicillin developed
1963	Gentamicin developed
1964	Cephalosporins developed

Newer Antibiotics

Further research took place during the 1960s, which led to the development of the second generation of antibiotics. Among these was methicillin, a semi-synthetic derivative of penicillin produced specifically to overcome the problem of penicillin resistance. Methicillin was hailed as a major breakthrough in the fight against bacterial resistance to penicillin, and scientists believed that they could now win this battle. Unfortunately, bacteria had the last word, and we now have bacteria that are resistant to methicillin.

Ampicillin is also a derivative of penicillin. It was developed to broaden the range of infections that penicillin could treat and has now replaced penicillin to a great extent. It is often the first choice in the treatment of a whole range of infections, including respiratory and urinary tract infections.

Amoxicillin is another widely used penicillin derivative. Like ampicillin, it has a broad range of activity, as it can treat both Gram-positive bacteria (those bacteria that retain the violet stain in a process called Gram's method or Gram's stain, used to classify bacteria—e.g., *Streptococcus spp.* and *Staphylococcus spp.*) and Gram-negative bacteria (those bacteria that do not retain the violet stain used in Gram's method—e.g,. *E. coli* and *Haemophilus influenzae*).

Gentamicin is in the same family of antibiotics as streptomycin (the anti-TB drug discovered in 1943). It is generally reserved for serious infections, as it can have severe toxic side effects on the ears and kidneys.

Fluoroquinolones

Recently, a new family of antibiotics called the fluoroquinolones has been developed by pharmaceutical laboratories. In addition to being effective against a broad range of bacteria, these antibiotics can reach a high concentration in the bloodstream when taken orally. This means that many more infections that may once have required a hospital stay can now be treated at home.

The fluoroquinolones are often used for cases in which long courses of antibiotics (weeks to months) are required. A whole range is now available, and are proving effective against bacteria that were once difficult to treat, such as the leprosy bacteria.

THE FUTURE

The search for new and more effective drugs, which began with Florey, Chain, and Waksman, continues today. The pace, however, has slowed remarkably, as it is now much more difficult for pharmaceutical companies to get approval for new drugs. The time delay between the discovery of an antibiotic in the laboratory and the approval to produce it commercially is so great that it has led some companies to abandon the marketplace completely. Companies involved in the search for new antibiotics are also finding it increasingly difficult to keep up with the pace at which bacterial resistance renders their findings useless.

CHAPTER 2

THE EFFECTS OF THE USE AND ABUSE OF ANTIBIOTICS

The Blind Leading the Blind

It is vitally important that we understand the mistakes we have made with antibiotics in the past so that these errors will not be repeated in the future. We need to be aware of where we have gone wrong and why.

Antibiotics are often prescribed for viral infections, such as colds, flu, glandular fever, herpes infections, and gastroenteritis. However, antibiotics have no role to play in the treatment of viral infections, as they neither kill nor stop the multiplication of viruses. Sometimes a viral infection can weaken the immune system, particularly in certain "at-risk" groups like the elderly, the very young, and post-surgery or other trauma patients. As a result, a viral infection may sometimes lead to the development of a secondary bacterial infection. It is this secondary bacterial infection that is often the reason why antibiotics are prescribed to patients with viral infections. Surely it would make more sense to wait to see if a bacterial infection develops and, if concerned, to boost the immunity of the person at risk first with natural means. Antibiotics should be used only if absolutely necessary in the prevention of a secondary bacterial infection

In 1976, an article entitled "What Do Patients Know About

Antibiotics?" was published in the *British Journal of Medicine* (Chandler and Dugdale). Of the people questioned in this study, 55 percent believed that antibiotics kill viruses, and only 46 percent believed that bacteria are killed by antibiotics. A staggering 75 percent believed that antibiotics should be given for colds and flu. Antibiotics were developed to treat bacterial infections, such as streptococcal sore throats. They should not be used for colds, flu, or other viral infections.

In very simple terms, bacteria can be described as single-celled organisms. They have a cell wall and a plasma membrane, and they contain genetic material. Antibiotics can kill bacteria by damaging different parts of the bacterial cell (for example, penicillin damages the cell wall). See Figure 2.1 below.

Viruses are not living cells. They have no cell wall and no plasma membrane. They are not able to carry out chemical reactions; therefore, they cannot reproduce or multiply by themselves. As viruses do not contain structures that antibiotics can attack, these drugs are useless against viruses. See Figure 2.2 on next page. Now you can understand why antibiotics are effective in the treatment of infections caused by bacteria, yet ineffective in the treatment of viral infections.

Antibiotics are also prescribed for relatively minor infec-

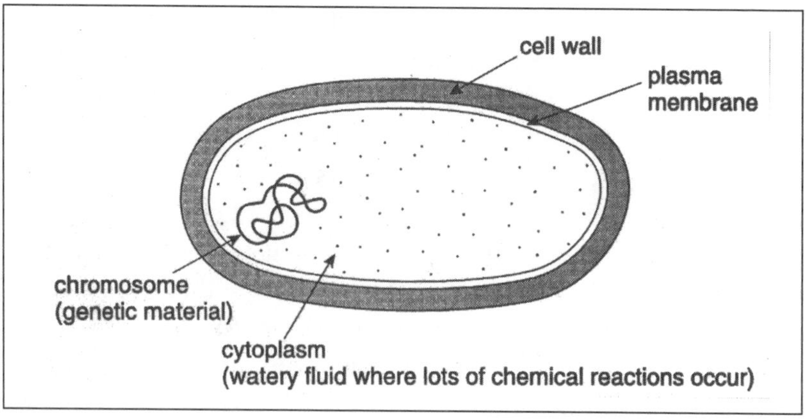

Figure 2.1 A bacterial cell (simplified)

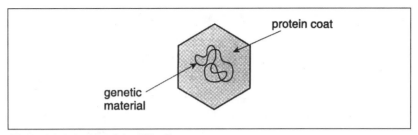

Figure 2.2 A virus (simplified)

tions that could be treated with simpler methods. Very often an infection requires no treatment at all, as your body will fight the infection on its own. But, if necessary, this fight can be assisted by natural means. It is important to let your body fight an infection, since this will allow you to build up a natural resistance to that particular infection. Only when the body is clearly not winning the battle should one intervene. Remember also, that many antibiotics do not kill bacteria outright as is commonly believed, they only stop their growth. Your immune system must do the rest.

Antibiotics are highly effective in treating bacterial infections. Unfortunately, they are being prescribed and taken far too carelessly. Patients often place pressure on their doctors to prescribe antibiotics; and the physicians, who should know better, are all too eager to comply; even when the cause of their patient's complaint has no relation to a bacterial infection. This carelessness, on the part of both doctor and patient, is the primary cause of the phenomenon of bacterial resistance that is now rendering antibiotics useless.

Antibiotics are potentially life-saving drugs. They represent a wonderful advance in medical science. When they first came on the scene, it was thought that the scourge of infectious disease would be gone forever and that humankind could live in a virtually infection-free world.

The truth has turned out to be rather different. Antibiotics are now being rendered useless by the very bacteria they were intended to destroy. Bacterial resistance is developing at an alarming rate. In fact, many hospital-based doctors are deeply concerned about the future.

I heard a group of doctors in New York speak about an epidemic of tuberculosis (TB) that is occurring in the United States. They were saying that this latest outbreak of TB is proving extremely difficult to treat because the "superstrain" of bacterium that causes it, *Mycobacterium tuberculosis,* is now resistant to most of the standard drugs (or multiresistant). Patients with this form of TB are presently untreatable. Doctors throughout Europe have also warned about the alarming increase in bacterial resistance to antibiotics and have urged general practitioners to be much more cautious in the way they prescribe antibiotic drugs. You, as a potential patient, can assist your doctor by discussing the alternatives with him/her and by asking for natural medicines.

The frightening truth of the matter is that the misuse of antibiotics has become a major public health hazard, and in the very near future, common infections may not respond to antibiotic treatment at all. Because of this overuse and abuse of antibiotics, we have lost sight of the fact that nature has its own methods of fighting back—producing multiresistant strains of bacteria. Ironically, it is to nature and natural medicine that we must look for a way out of this predicament. In this book, I want to show that there are effective, side-effect-free methods of treating infections and that these methods are also less likely to result in bacterial resistance in the years to come.

THE DANGERS OF EXCESSIVE ANTIBIOTIC USE

Overuse of antibiotics can cause many problems. Their use may even cause life-threatening problems for some. These problems will be discussed in this section.

Resistance

If antibiotics, such as penicillin, are used inappropriately or for a too short period of time, bacteria can develop resistance to them. Resistant strains are then able to counteract the effects of penicillin when they next come into contact with it. In this way, the drug begins to become ineffective. When many types of bacteria start to develop resistance to a drug, the drug begins to become useless. As a result of this, more powerful antibiotics have to be synthesized and manufactured. However, the pace at which bacterial resistance is developing is much faster than the pace at which drug companies are able to produce new antibiotics. The problem of bacterial resistance to antibiotics will be discussed at length in Chapter 3.

Allergic Reactions

Because of the overuse of antibiotics, allergic reactions to these drugs are increasingly common. It used to be that only 5 to 10 percent of people developed allergic reactions to antibiotics, mainly penicillin. Now, as more and more individuals are exposed to antibiotics more and more often, increasing numbers of people are developing allergic reactions to the drugs. These allergic reactions can range from a skin rash to edema (tissue swelling), to anaphylactic reactions, including bronchospasm (constriction of the airways) and shock. These reactions are not limited to the use of the penicillin group of antibiotics, either. They may occur also as a result of the use of the cephalosporins and tetracyclines.

Intestinal Problems

Antibiotics such as tetracycline and amoxicillin can disturb the intestinal bacteria, especially the "good," healthy bacteria, such as *Lactobacillus acidophilus* and *Bifidobacterium bifidus*. This disruption can lead to intestinal problems, such as diarrhea, flatulence, and abdominal distention (bloating). There is now evidence to suggest that disturbances of the intestinal bacteria may play a part in the development of bowel disorders, such as ulcerative colitis and cancer of the colon.

Another problem that can result from the disturbances of

intestinal bacteria is the overgrowth of yeast and fungi in the bowel, which leads to intestinal candidiasis. This is now a major problem in the Western world and coincides with the overuse of antibiotics. Candidiasis used to be a disease seen only in people whose immunity was compromised, for example, in babies whose immunity is still developing, in the elderly whose immunity is in decline, and in patients whose immunity has been suppressed for some reason, such as the long-term use of steroids. In the 1990s, intestinal candidiasis is affecting all age groups and all types of people. This concerns me, as it suggests that people's immunity is threatened.

Natural Alternatives to Antibiotics at Work

Sarah, a 6-year-old girl, had been suffering from abdominal pain and loss of appetite for three months. Prior to the onset of these symptoms, she had received four courses of antibiotics for ear infections that were very resistant to treatment. I diagnosed her as having intestinal dysbiosis (a disturbance in the bacterial population of the bowel). I altered her diet to exclude sugar and processed foods, and to include live yogurt and whey. I also gave her appropriate homeopathic remedies. Not only did her abdominal pain disappear and her appetite improve, but her ear infections disappeared as well.

This case is typical of many children who have been given one or more courses of antibiotics, especially broad-spectrum antibiotics like tetracycline and amoxicillin. Antibiotics can disturb the "good" bacteria that line the digestive tract. These bacteria manufacture a number of vitamins that the body needs for good health.

Depressed Immunity

Antibiotics may also have a suppressive effect on the immune system. Certain antibiotics, including tetracycline and the sulfonamides, can inhibit the activity of the white blood cells, which engulf and destroy bacteria. Other antibiotics are known to inhibit antibody production, thus lowering immunity (Hauser and Remington, 1982). Antibiotics have also been shown to increase the likelihood of recurrent infections. Studies published in 1974 (Diamont and Diamont) and more recently in 1991 (Cantekin et al.) have shown that children with earaches who received antibiotics, especially in the first few days, were much more likely to develop recurrent ear problems than those in whom treatment was delayed or to whom a placebo was given. In conventional medical circles, it is now widely accepted that doctors should either delay treatment of earaches or not treat them at all.

This documentation supports other evidence that shows that antibiotics can indeed suppress one's natural immune response to an infection and can set up a situation in which the infection recurs.

THE DANGERS OF THE USE OF SPECIFIC ANTIBIOTICS

In addition to the general problems that overuse of antibiotics may cause, such as bacterial resistance and allergic reactions, the use of certain individual antibiotics can also be dangerous due to their specific actions in the body.

Chloramphenicol

It is not uncommon for chloramphenicol to reduce the white blood cell count, particularly the type of white cell that fights bacteria invading the body—granulocytes. In rare cases—approximately one in 100,000—it can cause death by suppressing bone marrow function. It has been taken off the market in Europe and North America, although it is still used in many African countries.

Tetracyclines

There are several tetracyclines, including demeclocycline, doxycycline, minocycline, oxytetracycline, and tetracycline. As discussed in Chapter 1, they can damage the growing bones and teeth of fetuses and children below the age of seven. Such reactions occur because tetracyclines bind to calcium phosphate, thus allowing the drug to be absorbed by bones and teeth. This damages the dental enamel of the tooth with pitting, causes yellow/brown discoloration of the teeth, and increases susceptibility to dental cavities.

Tetracyclines are known to decrease the levels of some of the B vitamins in the body by disturbing their absorption in the bowel. They can also disturb the bacterial flora of the bowel. In addition, tetracyclines can cause diarrhea, especially after prolonged use. Less commonly, they can increase the pressure around the brain in a condition called benign intracranial hypertension.

The tetracyclines are potentially quite damaging antibiotics. They are often prescribed for the long-term treatment of teenage acne and are used for three to six months, and in some cases twelve months. It worries me that people are taking this type of antibiotic for such long periods of time.

Aminoglycosides

Included in this group of antibiotics is the anti-tuberculosis drug streptomycin, as well as gentamicin, kanamycin, tobramycin, neomycin, and amikacin. They are commonly used to treat infections where the invading bacteria cause urinary tract infections, peritonitis, and wound infections after bowel surgery. This particular group of antibiotics is quite toxic, as the drugs it contains can cause damage to the auditory nerve and so lead to deafness. The drugs in this group are also capable of damaging the kidneys and causing skin rashes and drug-induced fevers.

Sulfonamides

Sulfonamides include sulfacytine, sulfadiazine, sulfamethiazole, sulfamethoxazole, and sulfisoxazole. They can cause some serious side effects, including allergic reactions of many kinds (such as skin rash, fever, hepatitis, low white cell count, and aplastic anemia), diarrhea, and the formation of crystals in the urine. Sulfonamides are also known to cause pancreatitis and diabetes mellitus. Less serious side effects include malaise, headache, nausea, and vomiting, but these are usually transient.

ANTIBIOTIC USE PRECAUTIONS

Sometimes it may be necessary to take antibiotics. However, there are a number of steps you can follow to offset the negative effects of antibiotics and to maximize their effectiveness.

- Take live yogurt or other bacterial supplements, such as acidophilus capsules, with the antibiotic to prevent damage to the intestinal bacteria, which are important for a healthy bowel. When taking tetracyclines, however, be sure to use acidophilus capsules instead of yogurt because tetracyclines can bind to the calcium in dairy products, inhibiting calcium's absorption across the intestinal wall into the bloodstream.

- Use an immune booster to assist your body's immune response to the infection, as there is some evidence that suggests that antibiotics can suppress different parts of the immune system. Substances that boost immunity are discussed in Chapters 5 and 7.

- Take vitamin C along with an antibiotic, as vitamin C is known to increase the blood levels of certain antibiotics, thus making them more effective. I recommend a dose of 2,000 to 3,000 milligrams daily.

- Take the antibiotic for the entire prescribed period, as stop-

Natural Alternatives to Antibiotics at Work

Gerard was 7 years old and was suffering from recurrent ear and chest infections when his mother brought him to see me. His doctor had treated him with antibiotics each time he had an earache or a chest infection. Gerard's mother handed me a list of the antibiotics used and the dates they were prescribed. It is a good idea to keep such a record of the drugs that you have been prescribed. Here is the list.

Dates	Prescription
02/11/1993	Distaclor*
03/18/1993	EryPed (erythromycin ethylsuccinate)
05/17/1993	Augmentin (amoxicillin/clavulanate potassium)
05/30/1993	Septrin*
06/10/1993	Distaclor*
07/10/1993	Septrin*
07/15/1993	Augmentin (amoxicillin/clavulanate potassium)
09/01/1993	Augmentin (amoxicillin/clavulanate potassium)
09/10/1993	Augmentin (amoxicillin/clavulanate potassium)
09/27/1993	Distaclor*
12/23/1993	Augmentin (amoxicillin/clavulanate potassium)
01/04/1994	Septrin*
02/24/1994	EryPed (erythromycin ethylsuccinate)
02/27/1994	Distaclor*

* United Kingdom brand name.

That makes fourteen antibiotics given to a young child within a twelve-month period. This is frightening, but not the worst case I've seen. When I sent Gerard for testing, he had gross disturbance of his bacterial flora, as well as pancreatic damage. A change in diet, homeopathic medicines to boost his immunity, high-dose vitamin C, and live yogurt helped this child enormously. Since coming to see me, he has not needed another antibiotic, and the infections have ceased. This is the beauty of natural medicine. It is possible to help many people by getting them off conventional drugs and using safe alternative medicines.

Gerard's case history illustrates a prescribing pattern that is doing immense damage not only to patients who have to suffer the side effects of these drugs, but also to the medical profession, whose credibility is being undermined. That such a quantity of drugs can be prescribed to a young child is shocking, and it clearly highlights the futility of continuing to educate doctors in drug therapy alone. It is imperative that they be trained in the use of natural medicines. Interestingly, most medical students and doctors would favor such training. With your help, it can happen.

ping before the course has been completed will encourage the development of bacterial resistance and make a recurrence of the disease more difficult to treat.

- Insist on knowing all of the side effects before agreeing to use an antibiotic. Your doctor or pharmacist should be able to assist you in this regard.

Antibiotics should be used as the last resort, not the first. This book will describe methods that can be used in the initial stages of infection. If these measures fail, there may then be a need for antibiotics. In this way, antibiotics will become the exception rather than the rule and bacterial resistance will become less of a problem.

CHAPTER 3

BACTERIAL RESISTANCE TO ANTIBIOTICS

Taking the Intelligence but Leaving the Wisdom

As multiresistant bacteria continue to multiply and develop, the medical community finds itself faced with more and more potentially untreatable diseases. Part of the blame for this phenomenon is to be placed on the medical community itself. Over-prescription of and misuse of antibiotics—attempting to treat viral infections with antibiotic drugs for example—continues to contribute to the development of increasingly virulent bacteria.

This chapter addresses several issues surrounding bacterial resistance. In addition to a general discussion of the problem of resistant bacteria and the ways in which such a phenomenon may affect us, this chapter explains how and why bacteria develop resistance and discusses alternatives that may reverse this trend.

BACTERIAL RESISTANCE—THE PROBLEM

Even during the early stages of antibiotic development, it was clear that some bacteria could survive and multiply in the presence of antibiotics. These bacteria had acquired resistance to the effects of those antibiotics.

In an interview with *The New York Times* in 1945, Alexander Fleming warned that the misuse of penicillin could lead to the selection and multiplication of mutant forms of resistant bacteria. He also predicted that this problem of resistance would worsen if penicillin was made available in oral form, if inadequate doses were given, if a course of treatment was not completed, or if people were given too long a course of penicillin. Just how serious is this antibiotic-resistance problem, though?

In the early 1980s, a number of hospitals in Melbourne were plagued with infections that were resistant to almost all known antibiotics. The organism causing the problem, which resulted in the deaths of a number of hospital patients, was *Staphylococcus aureus*. This situation represents the gravest of resistance problems. It raised such fears among hospital workers that many of them wore masks at work. The bacteria were resistant not only to antibiotics but also to antiseptics, making them virtually impossible to kill. Only one antibiotic remained effective—vancomycin, a drug that is both expensive and toxic. Doctors had no alternative but to use it. In this way, the hospital infections were eventually brought under control.

It was a close call for Melbourne. What if resistance to vancomycin had developed? How would such a hospital-based infection have been treated? Would it really have become untreatable?

That was in the 1980s. Today, vancomycin resistance is indeed a reality, but it occurs in a different group of bacteria—*Enterococci*. We know, however, that these bacteria are able to transfer their resistance to *Staphylococcus aureus*, the organism that causes hospital-based infections. This means it is only a question of time until resistance to vancomycin occurs in *Staphylococcus*. Then, hospital infections, such as those in Melbourne, really will be impossible to treat with antibiotics.

So it is clear that we are facing a potentially disastrous situation. An infection that is untreatable by present means is now a real possibility. It is only a matter of months, or a year or two at most, according to some microbiologists.

WHY DO BACTERIA DEVELOP RESISTANCE?

The problem of widespread bacterial resistance is one that we have brought upon ourselves. Bacteria's reasons for developing resistance are simply a matter of the organisms' drive to survive. However, through our excessive use of antibiotics, we have exacerbated the need of the bacteria to fight for life to the point that the existence of bacterial resistance has become worrisome.

Bacterial resistance to antibiotics is not a new phenomenon; it has been around for as long as bacteria themselves, but at a very low level. We can see this in soil, for example, where fungi and bacteria coexist. This coexistence is not entirely peaceful, though. In fact, fungi and bacteria battle with each other for space and resources in the soil. Fungi compete with bacteria in the soil by producing antibiotics. (You may remember that many antibiotics were originally isolated from soil samples containing fungi.) In order to survive, bacteria devised a means of protecting themselves against these natural antibiotics; they developed resistance. So resistance is a natural survival mechanism.

But if resistance to antibiotics has always existed, why has it now become so widespread? And why is it such a danger? The answers to these questions lie in the way we have approached the use of commercial antibiotics. We have overused them in some instances and underused them in others. We have used them inappropriately in still other circumstances. In general, we have grossly misused them, and through this misuse, we have encouraged the never-ending development of resistance in bacteria.

I cannot overstate how important diet is, especially for those of us living in modern cities. It is easy to end up eating

Natural Alternatives to Antibiotics at Work

John was the financial director of a large computer software company. He had recurring symptoms of tiredness and a sore throat on and off for more than a year. A friend of his was a pharmacist, so, to save time and money, John got antibiotics directly from his friend and treated himself. By the time he sought medical help, he had taken seven different courses of antibiotics in the space of twelve months. His symptoms were not only no better; they were now persistent, and it was very difficult to keep working.

This man was too busy to seek medical help early on. Self-treatment seemed the best solution at the time. Self-medication with potentially harmful drugs only encourages the development of bacterial resistance. It can also cause long-term illness. Don't put pharmacists in the difficult position of having to diagnose and treat. The same applies to homeopathic pharmacists. Consult your doctor.

Simply by following a prescribed course of homeopathic medicines (to boost John's immune system and to undo some of the harmful effects of the antibiotics), altering his diet, and following high-dose vitamin C and live yogurt regimens, John was able to overcome his fatigue. The sore throats are now a thing of the past.

a very unnatural, highly processed diet. Then, when the inevitable occurs and the body starts to break down, we reach for unnatural medicines to treat it.

It is not only doctors and patients who are at fault when it comes to over-prescribing antibiotics; pharmacists and governments are too. In many developing countries, antibiotics are freely available without a prescription. This leads to their misuse, thereby encouraging the development of resistance.

While working in Africa, I saw a situation in which drugs, sent by an aid agency to assist a particular hospital, were being sold openly in the marketplace to anyone who had the money to purchase them. I have also seen cases where members of hospital staff have been caught stealing antibiotics, which they intended to sell to the local people as a way of boosting their income. But the problem is even more widespread than this.

Antibiotics have been used in animal feeds for quite a long time. Livestock—cattle and pigs in particular—are given large amounts of antibiotics as growth enhancers and to treat specific infections. These animals (and their products) end up as food in our supermarkets, either as meat or as dairy products, like cheese and milk.

The bacteria in these animals tend to be multiresistant—that is, they have resistance to many antibiotics at the same time. This multiresistance can be passed on to humans through direct contact with the animals, through contaminated food, or via the soil (the feces of these animals form part of the soil).

Interactions between humans and animals can alter the bacterial flora of each group. Flora is the bacterial population that lines the skin and cavities of the body, including the respiratory and digestive tracts. Resistant bacteria can spread from the animal to the human via feeding or handling. See Figure 3.1 on page 42.

Many of the antibiotics approved for use in animals are being administered by farmers without veterinary supervision. One farmer to whom I spoke was injecting a calf with penicillin as I interviewed him. He explained to me that the calf had a sprained ankle. He was able to get a number of antibiotics from the veterinary surgeon's office without consulting the veterinarian about the suitability of this treatment.

Over-the-counter sales of antibiotics for the farming community must be stopped. All antibiotics should be adminis-

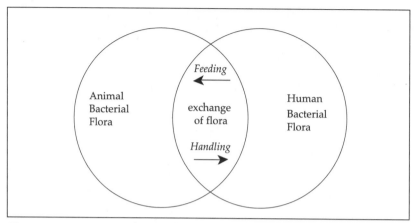

Figure 3.1 Bacterial exchange through human-animal interaction

tered by a veterinary surgeon and, as with humans, should be used as a last resort only. There are many excellent homeopathic remedies available for animals. The book *A Veterinary Materia Medica* by Dr. G. Mcleod is an excellent reference for anyone wishing to try alternative treatments for a variety of conditions affecting farm animals.

It is known that small amounts of penicillin and tetracycline can enhance the growth of livestock. Consequently, far greater amounts of antibiotics are given to commercial livestock to enhance growth than are used to actually treat infections. Administering even small amounts of antibiotics on a continuous basis can encourage bacterial resistance, as the bacteria develop their own means of overcoming the effects of the antibiotic instead of being killed by it. Using penicillin and tetracycline as growth enhancers has been stopped in Europe for the most part, but not in the United States and other parts of the world. This is clearly an issue that must be addressed globally.

Antibiotics are even used in our pets' food. One study has shown that 70 percent of dogs have in their feces a strain of multiresistant *E. coli*, a bacterium that is a normal constituent of the bowel in most animals, including humans (Monaghan et al., 1981). Some of the bacteria in the bowels of these dogs are resistant to two or more antibiotics. This may well be due to the fact that antibiotics are added to commercial dog foods as growth enhancers. And, as already discussed, even small amounts of antibiotics will encourage bacterial resistance.

Bacteria have the ability to develop resistance to almost any drug to which they are exposed. This resistance is now threatening our ability to treat infections, not only in humans, but also in animals. Using antibiotics in animal feeds to enhance the growth of livestock contributes greatly to the continuation and spread of resistance. The bacteria in the bowels of commercial animals (cattle, sheep, pigs), as well as in pets (cats, dogs), are resistant not just to one or two antibiotics but to many.

Antibiotic resistance is a worldwide problem that needs the cooperation of governments, doctors, pharmacists, veterinary surgeons, and farmers alike, as well as the education of the general public. In my opinion, it also requires the full support of the World Health Organization (WHO).

MULTIRESISTANT BACTERIA

In the late 1950s in a hospital in Japan, a very startling thing happened, alarming the whole scientific community—the birth of multiple drug resistance. In this hospital, a number of patients were suffering from *Shigella* dysentery. The bacteria causing this infection were resistant to tetracycline, the sulphonamides, streptomycin, and chloramphenicol. Multiple drug resistance was unknown prior to this. Now it suddenly sent shock waves across the world.

By 1966, a number of countries had reported multiple drug resistance. In one South African hospital, 50 percent of the *E. coli* bacteria isolated from the feces and urine of patients showed resistance to one or more antibiotics. Resistance information was carried by the plasmids (units of DNA that replicate within the cell independently of the chromosomal DNA) within the bacterial cell. These plasmids were transferred to other bacteria, making them multiresistant as well. In other words, the resistant bacteria share their ability to defeat antibiotics with other bacteria. They don't believe in being selfish!

Drug resistance has truly become a worldwide problem. Today, virtually the whole planet has a problem, to a greater or lesser extent, with antibiotic-resistant infections. This problem is not specific to the developing or developed parts of the world; it affects us all and, in a way, unites us.

Figure 3.2 shows the hospital laboratory report of a patient suffering from a urinary tract infection. As the report shows, the bacterium responsible for this infection was *E. coli* (a common cause of urinary infections). When a laboratory isolates a bacterium, it also tests to see which antibiotics will be most effective in treating the infection.

In the report, "S" means that the *E. coli* in the sample are sensitive to an antibiotic, so that antibiotics would effectively treat the infection. "R" means that the organism is resistant to an antibiotic, so that antibiotic would be ineffective as a treatment.

Look at the number of Rs in the report. This strain of *E. coli*

Dept. of Pathology
■■■■■■ Hospital

Date: 03-02-95
Doctor: Dr John Mc Kenna

Sample   : Urine   Patient ■■■■■■■■■■■■■

Investigation : Culture + Sensitivity

Report   : E. coli 10^5
                : Sensitivity

Amp/Amox	Velocef	Augmentin	Trimeth	Naldix	Nitro
R	R	R	R	R	R

Gentamycin	Sulpha	Amikacin	Netillin	Oflox	Ciproflox
R	R	R	R	R	R

Figure 3.2 Urine analysis of a patient with a urinary tract infection

is resistant to nine antibiotics. Truly multiresistant, it is sensitive to only three antibiotics, namely netimicin, ofloxacin, and ciprofloxacin. These drugs are rarely used to treat this condition.

A report like this, which indicates resistance to a large number of antibiotics, is very alarming. Furthermore, it is not uncommon. Soon, I expect to see strains of *E. coli* that can be treated only with one antibiotic. Not long after that, there will be strains of it that are untreatable altogether.

It is interesting to note that the patient referred to above is the wife of a commercial dairy farmer. This pattern of multiresistance is more common in patients from a farming background, probably because of the use of antibiotics in animals.

HOW DO BACTERIA DEVELOP RESISTANCE?

The mechanism by which bacteria overcome antibiotics, so-called "magic bullets," is fascinating. One can only be in awe of these changeable and resilient organisms and the ways in which they are able to overcome our efforts to kill them.

In a sense, it is our own narrow thinking and arrogance about nature—believing that we can control nature by killing off what we think is unnecessary or harmful—that have brought us to this deadly impasse. It is intriguing to think that we cannot control infectious diseases, but that they, in fact, have the potential to control us. They may even wipe us out!

Our limited thinking and our lack of awareness of nature are now forcing us to view things differently. We must accept that even pathogenic (disease-causing) bacteria have a positive and important role to play in nature. We don't have to understand what this role is; we need only respect it. Respect is the key to solving the problem of antibiotic resistance.

The health-care practitioners in underdeveloped countries seem to employ this respect. Many seem to have an understanding of the interconnectedness of all living things, and so are always attempting to work with nature by obeying its laws. They do not see themselves as different from, or better than, the rest of nature. Western civilizations, on the other hand, tend to see humans as all-important, as separate in some way and, therefore, able to rise above nature and control it. Simple single-celled organisms called bacteria have taught us the folly of our ways. Not only can they evade our magic bullets, but their ability to do so can also teach us a very valuable lesson. We all need to learn this lesson and to the shift our thinking away from control—control of nature, control of people, control of land—towards living in harmony with nature.

There will be more about our need to be in tune with nature later. For the moment, let's examine the ways in which bacteria are able to fight back.

Spontaneous Mutations

Bacteria have been able to survive over the centuries through a process known as spontaneous mutation. Every so often, genetic material mutates, or changes, and produces a gene that can help the bacteria to survive in the face of any toxic material in its environment, including antibiotics. At low levels of antibiotic usage, this is all that is necessary for survival. The presence of an antibiotic kills off the bacteria that are susceptible to it. This leaves behind those bacteria that possess genetic material which has mutated in such a way as to make them impervious to the antibiotic. These impervious bacteria, then, are left alive to reproduce. The gene for antibiotic resistance is passed on from one generation of antibiotic-resistant bacteria to the next. As those bacteria that are sensitive to antibiotic die, they leave behind a bacterial population that is composed of nothing but the initially rare antibiotic-resistant bacteria.

In the 1940s, Sir Alexander Fleming, a Scottish biologist, noticed such mutants in his experiments and warned of them. He predicted that the more widespread the use of antibiotics, the more widespread and more numerous these mutant forms would be. How right he was! Through spontaneous mutation, the genes of bacteria can adapt, enabling them to survive in a hostile environment. This is quite amazing. It shows how a change in the environment can cause unseen changes in the world of bacteria.

Plasmids

Ubiquitous use of antibiotics has led to bacteria becoming even more adaptable. They developed new, improved survival mechanisms in the form of plasmids. I first learned of plasmids in the Moyne Institute in Trinity College, Dublin, over twenty years ago. Little did I know then about the importance plasmids would assume in later years, especially in my own work.

Plasmids are self-duplicating mini-chromosomes, or extra bits of genetic material, that exist in a bacterial cell. They are independent of the chromosomes. Sometimes a plasmid mutates spontaneously, and it is from this mutation that an antibiotic-resistant gene arises. The plasmids containing the mutated gene now carry new information about how to survive in the presence of a previously deadly substance. In this way, they are able to help bacteria to adapt faster than ever to the changes going on around them. While we were making antibiotics widely available and patting ourselves on the backs for our wonderful scientific advances, bacteria were busy developing more efficient means of protecting themselves.

Plasmids are in a constant state of change. They are continually losing genes that are no longer of use to the survival of the cell and, at the same time, acquiring new genes. The environment dictates and selects which genes are of value and need to be retained, and which cells are no longer necessary for the cell's survival.

Through our misuse of antibiotics, we have ensured the development of plasmids and their continued importance.

The main function of plasmids is to prevent bacteria from being killed by antibiotics. Plasmids were unknown until the 1970s, when resistance became a major problem. They began to ring the death knell for penicillin and warned of what was to come.

A unique characteristic of plasmids is that they can be transferred from one bacterial cell to another and from one species of bacterium to another. This allows bacteria to become resistant to a drug very quickly. See Figure 3.3 below.

Transposons

There seems to be no limit to what bacteria will do in their war against antibiotics. If producing plasmids was not enough, bacteria have now developed transposons that transfer such properties as antibiotic resistance between genetic materials. Transposons are even smaller pieces of DNA (or genetic material) than plasmids. As the name suggests, they are able to jump from one piece of genetic material to another (transposition). They can jump from a plasmid to a chromosome or vice versa. Each transfer rearranges the DNA of the cell that the transposon comes to rest in. In this way, they can easily transfer resistance genes within a bacte-

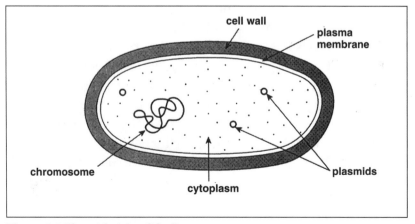

Figure 3.3 Plasmids (simplified)

rial cell or from one bacterial cell to another. This is an even faster and more efficient way of spreading resistance genes among a population of bacteria. Spontaneous mutations, the production of plasmids, and the development of transposons are the main methods bacteria employ to survive in the presence of antibiotics. These are the mechanisms that have led to the epidemics of bacterial resistance that currently plague many modern hospitals.

DID WE CREATE ANTIBIOTIC RESISTANCE?

To answer this question, we must visit the more remote peoples of this planet and see if they, too, carry bacteria that have antibiotic-resistant genes.

Studies have been performed on the Bushmen tribes of southern Africa. These people have little contact with the Western world and would never have taken antibiotics. The bacteria in stool samples from these people show very low, but detectable, numbers of resistant bacteria. The same result has been found in other studies of remote tribes in different parts of the world.

Among the Kalahari Bushmen, approximately one in fifty bacteria carry a resistance gene, whereas in European people, twenty-five out of fifty bacteria carry a resistance gene (see Figure 3.4 on page 50).

So, we did not create bacterial resistance. What we have done is encourage the development of resistant and multiresistant bacteria. In fact, we have unwittingly allowed these bacteria to flourish and prosper.

THE EFFECTS OF RESISTANCE

Bacterial resistance affects us all. However, the results of its existence are not entirely bad.

As with all situations in life, we can choose to view things negatively or positively. The negative way of viewing resistance is evident in the media. The problem of resistance is por-

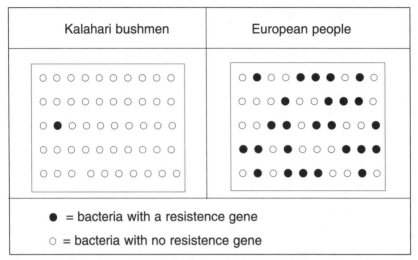

Kalahari bushmen	European people

● = bacteria with a resistence gene

○ = bacteria with no resistence gene

Figure 3.4 Bacterial resistance before and after antibiotic use (stool sample analysis)

trayed as a plague that can wipe out the whole of humanity in a short space of time. This may not be untrue, but if we created the problem, we can surely solve it too.

The more positive way of viewing resistance is to see it as a blessing in disguise. It is a blessing because it makes us stop and think. It makes us become more responsible for our actions (for example, not using an antibiotic as a quick fix if you have a cough or a cold). It is forcing all of us to educate ourselves not just about antibiotics but about the harmful effects of all drugs. It is asking us to make choices about our lifestyles. In more subtle ways, this problem of resistance is challenging our view of ourselves and our world, since we are finding it harder to view ourselves as superior to single-celled bacteria or as separate from them. It challenges our concept of control not just of nature but of many things in our lives.

Earlier in this chapter, you saw a hospital laboratory analysis of a urine sample. It showed that the strain of *E. coli* present in the sample was resistant to most antibiotics. I treated this patient with cranberry juice, which has been shown in a number of studies to be effective in the treatment of urinary tract infections; a complex homeopathic remedy containing echinacea; and high-dose vitamin C therapy. A repeat urine culture two weeks later showed no growth of *E. coli*. The infection had responded.

Resistance to antibiotics is a major public health problem. It is threatening our ability to fight even common infections like tonsillitis, ear infections, and urinary tract infections. Because it is such a massive problem, global in its dimensions and not well understood by the public, an organization called the Alliance for the Prudent Use of Antibiotics has been established in the United States to address the issue. The main aims of this organization are to encourage people to take a more responsible approach to the use of antibiotics and to promote the improved use of antibiotics through communication of research information from different countries around the world. It also seeks to educate people: doctors, patients, veterinary surgeons, farmers, pharmacists, pharmaceutical companies, and lay people alike. This kind of international cooperation involving all those interested in the use of antibiotics is absolutely necessary.

CAN BACTERIAL RESISTANCE BE OVERCOME?

Plasmids and transposons allow those bacteria that contain them to survive in the presence of an antibiotic; hence, survival of the fittest is clearly at work. But if a bacterial cell contains one or more plasmids (and/or transposons), this is disadvantageous to its survival in two ways. First, carrying this extra genetic material consumes a lot of the bacterial cell's energy, so less energy is available for its growth or reproduction. Second, the bacterial cell is less virulent with these passengers. One microbiologist has described multiresistant bacteria as "cripples."

So carrying resistance genes has both advantages and disadvantages for a bacterial cell. We are constantly pressuring bacteria to carry resistance genes through our misuse of antibiotics. If this pressure is removed by not using an antibiotic at all for a period of time, bacteria start to lose their plasmids/transposons and return to their original state.

In one hospital in Southern Africa, the doctors had a problem with bacterial resistance to an antibiotic called gentamicin. The doctors stopped prescribing gentamicin for a time, substituting a less common antibiotic instead. After a period of five years, the particular bacteria whose antibiotic resistance had been troubling them (*Klebsiella pneumonia*, which can cause lung infections) lost its resistance genes and once again became sensitive to gentamicin. Gentamicin, therefore, became useful again.

This suggests that a more prudent approach to the use of antibiotics will indeed result in bacterial changes. These changes will lead to reduced bacterial resistance and a return to their natural state of susceptibility to antibiotics. This is a beautiful example of the balances that work within nature.

CHAPTER 4

THE TREATMENT OF CHILDHOOD INFECTIONS

Antibiotics—the Exception, Not the Rule

Each year in the United States over $500 million worth of antibiotics are prescribed to treat one single problem—earache in young children. The prescribing of antibiotics for childhood infections has increased alarmingly over the past twenty years. Reread the case history in the Introduction to remind yourself of the ways children are being treated. This excessive prescribing of antibiotics costs a great deal, not only in financial terms but also in human terms.

In this chapter, I will discuss many common childhood infections and their appropriate treatments. Many are viral and do not require antibiotics. Many can be treated using alternative medicines. I shall deal only with the more common childhood infections, including those of the upper respiratory tract, the lower respiratory tract, the intestines, and the urinary tract. I shall also point out situations where an antibiotic may, in fact, be required.

UPPER RESPIRATORY TRACT INFECTIONS

Fifty percent of all infections in children are in the upper respiratory tract. These include infections of the nasal passages, throat, and ears. Upper respiratory tract infections, such as colds, flu, and runny noses, are viral; and antibiotics have no part to play in their treatment. Even if the discharge from the nostrils is yellowish or greenish, swabs consistently show no bacterial growth. If in doubt, have a nasal swab done by your family doctor, as this will show whether the infection is bacterial or not.

Antiviral measures include homeopathic remedies, nutritional and herbal enhancement of the immune system, and the use of vitamin C and, in some cases, zinc. (You will learn more about antiviral measures in Chapters 5 and 6, which deal with herbal medicine and homeopathy.)

I have found that children who do not respond to antiviral measures frequently have an allergy or intolerance to one or more foods—most commonly dairy products or sugar, which are mucus-forming foods. If an allergy or intolerance to a specific food is suspected, it is essential to avoid that food during treatment.

Middle Ear Infections

There are two situations that sometimes warrant the use of an antibiotic. The first of these is acute otitis media, or a middle ear infection. Somewhere between 30 and 50 percent of these infections—the literature seems to vary about the exact percentage—are bacterial. Most commonly, they are caused by *Streptococcus pneumoniae*.

A middle ear infection is marked by a severe earache. The inflamed eardrum may bulge. If it ruptures, there may be a discharge that starts out bloody, then changes to a clear fluid, and then changes to pus. Temporary hearing loss may occur. Young children may experience a high fever, nausea and vomiting, and diarrhea.

With middle ear infections, the recommendation is to wait a few days before taking an antibiotic, and in many cases to use no antibiotic at all. Scientists have recently established a link between an allergy to dairy products and recurrent ear infections. This possibility should be checked before using an antibiotic (Schmidt, 1990).

Researchers have also shown that many children with earaches for whom antibiotics are being prescribed actually have no bacterial infection in the middle ear. Other possible causes of earache include a viral infection; a blockage of the eustachian tube, the tube that connects the throat and middle ear; and an infection of the lining of the ear canal.

If an antibiotic is necessary, studies have shown that short courses of antibiotic treatment are just as effective as longer ones. For example, two-, four- and five-day courses of treatment are equally as effective as a ten-day course. In addition, delaying treatment for a day or two and using only painkillers will show if an antibiotic is really necessary.

Using antibiotics in the treatment of earache can predispose the patient to recurrent ear infections, especially with multiresistant bacteria. For example, children treated with amoxicillin have been shown to be two to eight times more likely to develop a recurrent infection.

Throat Infections

The other situation that may require an antibiotic is a bacterial sore throat, which is most commonly caused by *Haemolytic streptococci*. However, only about 30 percent of throat infections are bacterial. If your doctor prescribes an antibiotic for an ear or throat infection, make sure to use an immune stimulant along with it (see Chapter 5), as well as live yogurt to protect the intestinal flora (see Chapter 8). Some studies have shown that taking vitamin C along with an antibiotic can enhance the activity of the antibiotic. The duration of antibiotic treatment can be shortened as a result of this enhanced activity, thereby reducing its potential side effects. This is clearly an area that needs further research.

Symptoms of viral and bacterial throat infections are similar. Both produce a sore throat and inflammation of the mucous membrane lining the throat. However, a bacterial infection may produce a whitish membrane on the throat with a pus discharge, and it is more likely to produce a fever, enlarged lymph nodes, and an increased white blood cell count. Have your doctor perform a throat culture to be sure.

LOWER RESPIRATORY TRACT INFECTIONS

Children are also often plagued by lower respiratory tract infections, although these are not as common as upper respiratory tract infections. Antibiotics have a very limited role to play in the treatment of both upper and lower respiratory tract infections. Some children get recurrent upper or lower respiratory tract infections, or a mixture of the two. These are always viral. In some cases, they can be aggravated by environmental factors such as stress, a smoky atmosphere, or a damp house. There is no basis for the use of antibiotics in these cases; antiviral measures should be used.

Croup

Croup is a contagious infection of the upper and lower respiratory tracts that causes difficulty breathing, especially inhaling. The illness usually begins with cold-like symptoms, but breathing becomes more and more difficult, especially at night. It also produces a harsh, barking cough. Symptoms may improve during the day, only to worsen at night. With croup, 95 percent of infections are viral, usually caused by the para-influenza group of viruses, and antiviral measures should therefore be used. The other 5 percent of cases, however, tend to be bacterial, caused by *Haemophilus influenzae*. These bacteria can release toxins—substances that are poisonous to the body—which can make the child much more ill and can be life-threatening. If there is any suspicion that croup is bacterial, the child should be admitted to a hospital.

The following are signs of bacterial croup:

- The child is very unwell.
- The child may have a muffled voice.
- The child cannot swallow saliva and drools.

Bronchitis and Pneumonia

Bronchitis is inflammation of the airways, usually caused by infection. Unlike cases that occur in adults, the majority of acute bronchitis infections in children are viral. A number of different viruses may be responsible for the infection, including respiratory syncytial virus, para-influenza virus, adenovirus, or rhinovirus. Again, antiviral treatment is what is needed here.

Initial symptoms mimic those of a cold. However, a cough that starts out dry but begins bringing up sputum develops. While other symptoms may disappear after a few days, the cough lasts for several weeks. Pneumonia may develop.

In the rare instances in which childhood bronchitis is bacterial, the infection is more serious and would most commonly be caused by *Streptococcus pneumoniae*, which can lead to pneumonia. If there are signs of a bacterial infection, some doctors admit the child to the hospital, which is probably the safest option; others prefer to treat the child at home.

Pneumonia is an infection of the small air sacs (alveoli) of the lungs, and the surrounding tissues. It is most often caused by bacteria, but can also be caused by viruses, fungi, and bacterialike organisms. Symptoms include a cough that produces sputum, chest pain, fever, chills, and shortness of breath. Streptococcal pneumonia can be treated with penicillin. Although *Streptococcus pneumoniae* is usually the cause of infection, it is important to consider the possibility of staphylococcal pneumonia, as this requires a rather different course of treatment. Many forms of staphylococcal pneumonia are resistant to penicillin, so oxacillin or nafcillin are the antibiotics of choice for the treatment of staphylococcal pneumonia. Pneumonia that is caused by other bacteria is very rare, except in those whose immunity is compromised.

Bronchitis or pneumonia is particularly severe and in need of prompt medical attention when the rate of breathing increases to over 60 breaths per minute in infants, over 40 breaths per minute in toddlers, and over 30 breaths per minute in school children; there is respiratory distress, such as gasping for air; there is cyanosis (the patient turns blue); and the pulse increases to over 180 beats per minute in infants, over 160 beats per minute in toddlers, and over 110 beats per minute in school children.

Asthma

There is little to no basis for using antibiotics with patients who have asthma, since it is not caused by bacteria. Sometimes an asthma attack may be precipitated by an infection, but, generally, this is a viral infection caused by such viruses as respiratory syncytial virus, rhinovirus, and para-influenza virus. Antiviral treatment is called for, not antibiotics.

OTHER CHILDHOOD INFECTIONS

In addition to infections of the respiratory tract, infections of the digestive and urinary tracts are also common in children. Below, just a couple of these infections are discussed, as they are the most common.

Gastroenteritis

Like most respiratory infections, 60 percent of all cases of gastroenteritis in children under the age of five are caused by a virus. If bacterial infection is suspected, stool cultures should be done. Only when the infection is proven to be bacterial should antibiotics be considered. However, even if the infection is bacterial, antibiotics may be the wrong form of treatment. In gastroenteritis, antibiotics can exacerbate the condition by worsening the diarrhea. They can also predispose the child to a widespread infection with *Candida spp.* or *Staphylococcus spp.*, both of which may be life-threatening. Without the use of antibiotics, most cases of gastroenteritis are self-limiting. The mainstay of treatment must always be rehydration, either orally or intravenously.

Urinary Tract Infections

In contrast to most respiratory and bowel infections, urinary tract infections (UTIs) are generally bacterial in nature. Because of this, antibiotics may have a role to play in their treatment. However, it is always better to use natural methods first. I have successfully treated many cases of UTI using only natural medicines. The case mentioned in Chapter 3, in which I used natural methods, including cranberry juice, to treat a UTI shows that in many instances, antibiotics are not necessary. If natural methods do not control the infection, then there is a place for antibiotics.

The cause of urinary tract infections is usually contamination of the vagina or urethra with feces from the bowel. The most common bacterium in urinary tract infections is *Escherichia coli (E. coli)*. All children under the age of five who have recurrent urinary tract infections should have an IVP (intravenous pyelogram) done. This involves injecting dye into one of the veins in the arm and taking X-rays of the urinary tract to screen for abnormalities. The most common abnormality detected is reflux of urine from the bladder back up into the ureter.

ILLNESSES THAT MAY NOT RESPOND TO TREATMENT

There may be factors, other than infection, that can explain why a child does not respond to treatment, either with conventional drugs, alternative medicine, or both. Below are five conditions worth keeping in mind.

Natural Alternatives to Antibiotics at Work

Sean was a 4-year-old boy who had had a persistent cough for more than three years. He developed the cough at the age of 6 months, shortly after vaccination with the DPT vaccine, which vaccinates against diphtheria, tetanus, and whooping cough. The cough was dry, came in bouts, got worse at night, and occasionally changed to a productive cough with yellow sputum. All investigations—chest X-ray, blood tests, sputum culture, and swabs—revealed no signs of illness. The child's diet was well-balanced and very healthy.

I treated this as a viral infection following vaccination and used an antiviral homeopathic medicine, high-dose vitamin C therapy, and an herbal immune enhancer called echinacea-baptisia compound. (See Chapters 5, 6, and 7 for more information on these treatments.) The cough began to improve and was gone within two weeks.

Sean's cough was due to a viral infection of the lower respiratory tract, and it responded very well to antiviral treatment. The fact that it began just after vaccination was interesting because I have seen many children react negatively to certain vaccines, particularly the *pertussis* (whooping cough) and the measles vaccines. In some children, these vaccines appear to suppress the immune system and allow a chronic infection to develop, as in Sean's case. When a child has a negative reaction to a conventional vaccine, I recommend that the child be treated homeopathically to undo the damage the conventional vaccine may have done to the body. I also recommend that such children be given homeopathic vaccines in the future to prevent another such occurrence.

There are three types of homeopathic vaccines. One is the use of 1 ml of a live virus (for example the measle virus) diluted in 99 ml of water. The solution is then diluted 30 times in 99 ml of water. This solution is given to the child to either undo some of the damage done by the conventional vaccine or to protect the child from developing the infection. A second homeopathic vaccine is the use of a homeopathic remedy to treat the symptoms commonly associated with a given infection. A third homeopathic vaccine is the use of a constitutional remedy, which strengthens the "constitution" of the patient. This makes the person less susceptible to infection.

It is not uncommon for conventional vaccines (especially the DPT and the measles-mumps-rubella vaccines) to cause difficulties. This is why many parents opt for the diptheria-tetanus vaccine, which excludes the whooping cough vaccine.

This case shows that it is relatively easy to treat both chronic and acute viral infections in young children. When a child does not respond to treatment, I refer the child for testing to determine whether or not other factors are involved in the infection—allergies; reactions to medicines or vaccines; poor nutrition; exposure to various pollutants, including heavy metals; parasites; less common infections, including tuberculosis; and so on. By conducting thorough tests, using both conventional and alternative medical techniques, I have been able to find the underlying cause in all cases. This is much better than treating the patient blindly, time and time again, in the hope that something will work. It does not make sense to keep a child on medication long-term. I believe it is much more fruitful to put time and effort into finding the underlying cause of a child's symptoms and to then treat that.

Tuberculosis

Tuberculosis is a contagious, potentially fatal bacterial infection. One infected with tuberculosis often feels only malaise and has a cough that may produce some green or yellow sputum. The amount of sputum increases as the disease progresses. Profuse cold sweats and shortness of breath are also common symptoms. The infection may also cause weight loss. Often, a child with tuberculosis is free of symptoms, and the disease is discovered only when a chest X-ray is performed. Fortunately, however, tuberculosis is not very common in the United States.

Cystic Fibrosis

Cystic fibrosis is a relatively rare condition affecting approximately 1 in 2,000 children. It is a hereditary disease that causes certain glands, particularly in the digestive tract and lungs, to produce abnormal secretions. Bronchial secretions block airways and make breathing difficult. The child may suffer from poor digestion and nutrient absorption. The illness may also be associated with poor weight gain, slowed growth, loose stools, and prolapse of the rectum. The majority of patients are diagnosed in infancy, but a significant number with mild symptoms are first diagnosed in later childhood. The diagnosis is made by finding high sodium and chloride levels in sweat.

Mycoplasmal Pneumonia

This affects children of school-going age, from about five to fifteen years old, and can cause a wide range of respiratory tract infections. It is caused by the bacterialike organism *Mycoplasma pneumoniae*. Children affected by the disease exhibit extreme fatigue, loss of appetite, a sore throat, and a persistent cough. There may be a fever as well. The symptoms slowly worsen and usually last for one to two weeks, although the fatigue may persist for several weeks. The diagnosis is often suspected after a chest X-ray and is confirmed by finding specific antibodies in the bloodstream.

Reduced IGA Levels

IGA is an antibody that protects the lining of the respiratory tract. Children with impaired immunity, or reduced IGA, fail to thrive and have loose stools. A blood test is sufficient to diagnose this condition. It is much rarer than any of the above.

Inhalation of a Foreign Body

Sometimes a child can inhale a small object into the airway. Babies and toddlers are most at risk for this occurrence, as they tend to put everything in their mouths. The foreign body may block the airway at any level. If it lodges in the lower airway, there will be no symptoms for a time, until part of the lung collapses or an infection develops. If an obstruction of the airway is suspected as the reason a cough or other symptom is unresponsive to treatment, chest X-rays, including X-rays from the side (lateral chest X-rays), should be carried out. However, translucent objects, such as a piece of hard candy, may not show up on an X-ray. In this case, bronchoscopy, passing a scope down into the airway in order to view its contents, may be necessary.

The above conditions are best treated with a combination of conventional and alternative medicines. In all of these cases, testing would be important in order to assess which medicines to use, what dosage to give, and how long the treatment period should be. Treatment should involve the cooperation of a pediatrician and a homeopathic doctor. The fifth condition, inhalation of a foreign body, should be treated in a hospital.

Most common childhood infections are viral. Whether discussing upper respiratory tract, lower respiratory tract, or bowel infections, the mainstay of treatment should be antiviral measures, not antibiotic!

For the treatment of viral infections:

- Boost the immune system. The subsequent chapters will provide you with information on how to do this.
- Take vitamin C. Suggested dosages are discussed in Chapter 7, which deals with nutritional supplements.
- Use antiviral homeopathic medicines. These are discussed in Chapter 6.

We live in a quick-fix, superficial society. We do not want to tolerate any pain or suffering. We want instant cures. The cost of not truly treating the cause of the pain or illness is acceptable, provided we don't have to suffer. The medical profession supports this attitude by prescribing pills to take away the illness—or so it would appear. I see many children with recurrent infections in whom the illness clearly is not being treated. They are being provided a quick-fix over and over again. No one benefits from this type of short-term, limited approach. The child does not get better, the parent becomes more anxious, and the doctor becomes increasingly frustrated, as there is a limit to the number of drugs a doctor can prescribe. Furthermore, society in general suffers as the problem of bacterial resistance continues to grow because of these prescribing practices.

The days of using antibiotics alone in the treatment of an infection are coming to an end. The need to rationalize the use of these drugs is urgent. It takes courage on your part to stop accepting antibiotics as the answer to all infections and to demand a broader approach that includes nutrition, nutritional supplements, and natural medicines, as well as comprehensive methods of testing that involve both alternative and conventional medical techniques.

The issue of the side effects associated with antibiotic use is also of major importance. The bulk of prescriptions for these drugs are for childhood infections, and the damage they are doing to young children concerns me greatly. I consider it important enough to write a separate book on this subject, as a body of interesting information regarding this subject is beginning to appear in the medical literature. That book will spell out the reality of using antibiotics and the negative effects they can have on the human body.

Meanwhile, please remember that in many cases, especially with childhood infections, antibiotics are being prescribed inappropriately. The most commonly prescribed drug in the United States is amoxicillin—an antibiotic. Other antibiotics also rank high on the list of most commonly prescribed drugs in the United States. Isn't it time we asked why such drugs rank top of the list?

In earlier chapters, I explained the problem of resistance to antibiotics and the urgent need to take action. I also showed that many infections, especially childhood infections, should not be treated with antibiotics. The majority of infections respond very well to natural medicines. I will discuss some of these natural medicines and how they work in the next few chapters. Let's begin by looking at herbal medicine.

Chapter 5

HERBAL MEDICINE

The Mother of All Medicine

Herbal medicine is the oldest and most tried and tested form of medicine. In a sense, it is degrading to refer to it as an alternative, as it forms the basis of all medicine: conventional drugs, homeopathic medicine, and Traditional Chinese Medicine, to name only a few. It is the original medicine, the mother of all remedies used today. Herbal medicine has been used by all cultures for centuries and is still the main form of medical treatment among 80 percent of the world's population. It is sad to hear some doctors describe herbal medicine as quackery, as many of the drugs commonly used today, such as quinine, reserpine, ephedrine, and ipecac, come directly from plants, and most synthetic drugs are based on chemicals extracted from herbs.

There are a number of plants that have strong antibiotic and immune-strengthening properties. Used correctly, these herbs form the basis of all natural antibiotics. It is fascinating to discover that many of the helpful chemicals in these plants are of little benefit to the plant itself. Many of these chemicals have been produced by the plants to assist the rest of nature. The beauty and wisdom of the natural world is astonishing!

This chapter discusses the art of natural medicine and its

ability to bring you closer to the natural world. It also includes a discussion of the differences between synthetic drugs and herbal medicine. Finally, you will find an in-depth discussion of various herbs that are used to treat infectious disease.

HERBS—LINKING YOU TO NATURE

All life on this planet depends on the sun. The sun provides us with light and heat energy. Plants use light energy to make food in an amazing process called photosynthesis. Photosynthesis is the process by which green plants, using the energy of sunlight, convert carbon dioxide and water into food for themselves. Oxygen is released as a by-product during this process. In addition to being vital for our survival by providing us with oxygen, photosynthesis beautifully exemplifies one of Albert Einstein's theories—that energy and matter are the same thing, and that one can be converted into the other.

While photosynthesis shows how energy can be converted into matter, there is another remarkable process that can convert matter—the plant's nutrients—back into energy. This process is called cellular respiration, where the cells of the body break glucose down to release energy. When we eat the plant, we ingest the food that it has manufactured for itself through the process of photosynthesis. This food is then broken down into smaller units, or digested, and eventually ends up being used in cellular respiration to provide energy for the body.

Figure 5.1 illustrates an important point—when you use herbs or plants for healing, you are part of an energy transfer and, therefore, part of nature. The energy in this example comes from the sun and flows through nature to you. When you use an herb, you are actually part of something much greater. You are linked to something happening millions of miles from Earth. This is why natural medicines are so wonderful to use—they work at various levels within you, not just the physical.

TAPPING INTO INSTINCT AND ANCESTRAL KNOWLEDGE

Modern conventional medicine is not the only way to treat an illness. If a dog has eaten meat that has gone bad, it will eat some couchgrass *(Agropyron repens)* to make itself vomit. It knows instinctively which plant to eat to treat itself. Those in cultures that practice only herbal medicine know which plants to use to cure different ailments based upon years and years of trial and error and knowledge that has been passed from generation to generation. Our ancestors had a similar wealth of knowledge that was also handed down from generation to generation. This wealth of knowledge must be respected. Science has tried to diminish its importance and to substitute analysis for intuition. We know instinctively what our bodies need to stay healthy. Trusting these instincts is not so easy, however. As children, we were not encouraged to be trusting of our intuition, so we find this very difficult to do as adults.

Natural medicine is more an art than a science. Doctors, therapists, and healers must have a well-developed sense of intuition to work in this area. The reverse is true of conventional medicine, which has allowed itself to become very scientific. A marriage of the two can result in a harmony between art and science, between intuitive ability and scientific skills.

A SAFER ALTERNATIVE TO SYNTHETIC DRUGS

In 1874, sodium salicylate (synthetic aspirin) was chemically synthesized in a laboratory for the first time. This led to a surge in the use of synthetic medicines and a decline in the use

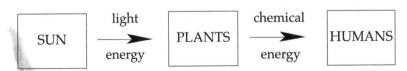

Figure 5.1 Energy transfer that occurs through the use of herbs.

of herbs. We assumed that all of our medicines could be produced in laboratories and that nature would become obsolete. Gradually, however, this assumption has been dispelled.

The thalidomide disaster in the late 1950s and early 1960s was a major warning sign of the dangers of using synthetically produced medicines. Thalidomide was given to pregnant women as a treatment for morning sickness, but it was soon linked to congenital defects in the unborn children. The children were born with flipperlike appendages in place of arms and legs. Another example of a dangerous synthetic medicine is Opren, an anti-inflammatory drug used to treat arthritis, which killed a number of patients suffering from that condition. Furthermore, in June of 1986, all children's medicine containing aspirin had to be taken off the market because a number of children had died from Reye's syndrome, a condition that causes brain and liver damage, as a result of aspirin use. The problem of side effects has considerably weakened the arguments in favor of using synthetic drugs. Justifiably, today most people are concerned about the use of conventional medicines.

Not all aspects of chemical analysis and laboratory research are negative, though. In fact, the scientific knowledge we have gained has been of considerable value. It has, for example, proven beyond doubt the claims made by ancient healers about certain plants. The shamans, traditional doctors of the North American Indians, have long claimed that plants such as *Echinacea purpurea* and *Baptisia tinctoria* (wild indigo) can be used to treat infections. Scientific researchers have isolated particular chemicals called glycoproteins and polysaccharides from these herbs and found that they both stimulate the immune system and damage invading bacteria. Hence, modern techniques have substantiated what "primitive" healers have been saying for some time—that these herbs are effective in the treatment of infections.

Scientists have also analyzed an herb called meadowsweet

(Filipendula ulmaria) and found that it contains a natural aspirin and can be used as a painkiller. The beauty of this analysis is that it has also shown that meadowsweet contains the substances tannin and mucilage, both of which act to protect the lining of the stomach. This means that meadowsweet does not irritate the stomach, a side effect often associated with synthetic aspirin. Remedies based upon chemicals will never compare with the beauty and intelligence of natural medicines. Daniel Mowrey's excellent book *The Scientific Validation of Herbal Medicine* should convince even the most skeptical reader of the validity of herbal medicine. Table 5.1, on page 72, briefly compares conventional and herbal medicine.

Unlike synthesized medicines that are designed to treat only the problem, herbal medicine can actually bolster your immune system, making you less vulnerable to disease from the start.

HERBS THAT FIGHT INFECTION

Over the centuries, a number of herbs have been used to fight many different types of infection. These herbs may still be used today as both effective and safe alternatives to synthetic antibiotics. I shall begin by discussing one of the most famous herbs of all, echinacea. The recommmend dosages for the discussed herbs are for adults. To determine the appropriate dosage for children between the ages of six and sixteen, place the child's weight in pounds in a fraction over 150 and give that fraction of the dosage to the child the same recommended number of times per day. For example, if the child is 50 pounds, give him or her 50/150 (or 1/3) of the adult dose.

Echinacea

Echinacea *(Echinacea purpurea)* is famous for its ability to fight infection and boost the immune system. It is one of the most commonly used herbs in the world, particularly in the United

States and Germany, although it is not as well known in other parts of Europe. This is probably because echinacea is indigenous to North America, where for centuries it has been used by the native North Americans in the treatment of infections, skin wounds, and snake bites. A German doctor, Dr. Meyer, learned about it from the Pawnee tribe in the late 1800s and used it to produce a medicine called Meyer's Blood Purifier. By the turn of the century, many doctors were using echinacea, and by 1907 it had become the most popular herb in medical practice. As a result of Dr. Meyer's influence, the

Table 5.1 Conventional Drugs Versus Herbal Medicines

Conventional Drugs	*Herbal Medicines*
Based on isolated chemicals.	Based on the whole plant.
Many may now be made synthetically.	All are natural.
Not part of the natural energy cycle and so are deficient in energy.	Are energy-rich, as they use the sun's energy.
Use unnaturally high concentrations of chemicals, which can disturb a natural system like the body and cause side effects.	Use natural substances and so are much safer for the body.
Are more dramatic in their action, as they enter the bloodstream rapidly.	Are slower to work.
Lower the vitality of the body and increase the work of elimination.	Enhance the vitality of the body by providing minerals and vitamins.

herb became popular in Germany, and today more than 250 medical products in Germany contain echinacea.

Echinacea is one of the most important natural remedies for treating both acute and recurrent infections. It is effective against a wide range of microbes, including many viruses, bacteria, and fungi. It can be used internally to treat infections anywhere in the body, and can also be used for external conditions as an ointment or salve. It is described as the herb that will convince even the most skeptical of physicians of the power of herbal remedies. As such, it has done much to convert many conventional doctors to natural medicine.

How Does Echinacea Work?

Echinacea stimulates the white blood cells that help to fight infections in the body. Recent research has shown that it enhances the activity of a particular type of white blood cells—macrophages. In December 1984, the medical journal *Infection and Immunity* reported that a particular glycoprotein (a carbohydrate-conjugated protein) in echinacea significantly increased the killing effect of macrophages on tumor cells.

What Is Echinacea Used to Treat?

Because echinacea can assist in the body's defenses, it helps to control viral, bacterial, and fungal infections. It is also used for skin wounds and can even be used to treat eczema.

Echinacea can be used to treat:

- Allergies.
- Bites and stings.
- Burns.
- Colds and flu.
- Ear infections.
- Eczema.
- Low white blood cell count.
- Sinusitis.

- Skin ulcers.
- Sore throats.
- Staphylococcal infections.
- Urinary tract infections.

How Is Echinacea Taken?

Echinacea is best taken as a concentrated liquid extract, or tincture. It is more easily absorbed into the bloodstream in liquid form, and it will have a longer shelf-life in this form. I find that I get much better results with it as an alcohol extract than in dry, capsule, or tablet form.

To treat an infection, take one-half to one teaspoon of echinacea as an herbal extract in liquid form three times daily for seven to ten days. Another method would be to take echinacea in homeopathic form. Take twenty drops as the first dose, and then take ten drops up to six times daily for two days. Then take ten drops three times daily for up to one week after overcoming the infection. For more serious infections, I recommend *Echinacea compositum*, a homeopathic medicine that will be discussed in Chapter 6. For more information on homeopathic remedies, see Chapter 6.

The quality and freshness of an herb is of great importance. I generally use the root of the plant *Echinacea purpurea*. In certain cases, I combine it with *Echinacea angustifolia*, as there is now evidence to suggest that the two are best used together to treat certain conditions. Echinacea in capsule or tablet form is used mainly by patients who cannot tolerate the taste of the liquid extract, but this is quite rare.

Occasionally, I use echinacea alone, but more often I combine it with other herbs. For example, in the treatment of sinusitis, I combine it with goldenseal or marshmallow. For certain respiratory tract infections, it is best combined with wild indigo. For immune enhancement, I combine it with astralagus, wild indigo, or myrrh; and for lymphatic drainage, I combine it with cleavers or pokeroot.

Is Echinacea Safe to Use?

Echinacea is generally recognized as one of the safest herbs. Many tests have shown it to be nontoxic, and in the last five years, I have not seen it produce any side effects. It should be noted, however, that echinacea should not be used by those with autoimmune disorders. In autoimmune disorders, the immune system, for some reason, begins to attack itself, and since echinacea is an immune system booster, it may only enhance this effect.

Wild Indigo

Wild indigo *(Baptisia tinctoria)* is another North American plant that has been used by the indigenous peoples for centuries. The Creek Indians, for example, used to give an extract of the root to children showing signs of infection, to help them fight it. Wild indigo was also used by other tribes, mainly for infections but also to treat wounds and bruises.

Wild indigo, also known as American indigo, false indigo, horsefly weed, indigo broom, yellow broom, and yellow indigo, is virtually unknown as a medicinal herb in Europe, although it has been used in German homeopathic medicine since the mid-1800s. Like *Echinacea purpurea*, the active constituents of wild indigo are in the roots. The chemicals that stimulate the immune system consist of glycoproteins and, to a lesser extent, polysaccharides. Wild indigo has antibiotic and immune-stimulating effects as well as anticatarrhal properties.

How Does Wild Indigo Work?

Wild indigo has an antibiotic effect on a wide range of microbes, including many bacteria and fungi. As such, it kills the microbe by preventing it from multiplying in the body. It also has an immune-enhancing effect, and some of the chemicals in wild indigo have a strong decongestant effect. It is interesting to note that many of the anti-infective herbs simultaneously stimulate one's immunity. This is the beauty of using natural remedies.

Taking wild indigo orally in the form of a tincture, a sort of liquid extract, can lead to a 30-percent increase in the number of white blood cells—the cells that fight infection—within two to three hours of taking the substance. This data is supported by further research from other studies. Using a homeopathic preparation of the herb, as described in Chapter 6, produces a similar result.

More recent research on wild indigo glycoproteins indicates that they appear to activate the lymphocytes, a particular type of white blood cell, the most.

What Is Wild Indigo Used to Treat?

Because of its antibiotic and decongestant effects, wild indigo is most useful in the treatment of infections of the respiratory tract. It is effective in the treatment of various acute and chronic infections of the sinuses, the lining of the nose, the tonsils, the throat, the lower respiratory tract, the larynx, the trachea, and the bronchi.

I have found it especially beneficial in the treatment of infections associated with the production of large amounts of mucus in the upper respiratory tract—the ears, nose, throat, and sinuses. I have also used it as a mouthwash to heal mouth ulcers and to treat gingivitis. Like echinacea, wild indigo can also be used externally. It can be applied as an ointment or salve to treat abrasions, skin infections, wounds, and sore nipples in breast-feeding mothers.

How Is Wild Indigo Taken?

As with echinacea, for maximum benefit, wild indigo is best used as a tincture. The recommended dosage for this form is two to four milliliters three times a day. It can, however, be used in powder, capsule, or tablet form. The roots of this herb are usually dug up in the autumn, cleaned, dried, and then chewed or ground up into a powder. It is used in this form to make a liquid extract that can be taken internally. It may also be used in a mouthwash when treating infections of the mouth. See your health-care practitioner for the recommended dosages for other forms of wild indigo and for the necessary duration of treatment for your illness.

The freshness of the herb is an important consideration. A liquid extract will have a much longer shelf-life—approximately one to two years—whereas the capsules or tablets have a much shorter period of usefulness. If using the latter, check the expiration date.

For the treatment of infections, I often combine wild indigo with echinacea or myrrh, as they are all immunity enhancers.

Is Wild Indigo Safe to Use?

Like echinacea, wild indigo has a wonderful safety record. It may even be given to very young children at the correct dosage. See the guidelines on page 71 to figure out the correct dosage for your child. It can be used with confidence for the above-mentioned infections in both adults and children. Large doses of the tincture, however, have caused poisoning.

Myrrh

Myrrh (*Commiphora molmol*) grows as a bush in the arid regions of Arabia, the Middle East, and northeast Africa. The people of these regions have been collecting the gum resin from this plant for centuries and have used it to treat a range of infections. The gum is often referred to as "gugal gum," and the plant is sometimes called Guggulu. The Arabs used it for stomach complaints and for respiratory infections—an arid climate is quite hard on the respiratory system!

How Does Myrrh Work?

Extracts from the plant have been shown to enhance phagocytosis (the bacteria-killing effect of white blood cells). As such, myrrh is effective at helping your body to fight a whole range of infections—viral, bacterial, and fungal. Like echinacea, recent research has indicated that it also has a direct antimicrobial effect.

What Is Myrrh Used to Treat?

Of the herbs discussed so far, myrrh is the strongest agent for treating skin infections. It can be used to treat abscesses, boils, sores, and wounds. Internally, myrrh can be used to treat asthma, bronchitis, colds, flu, sinusitis, sore throats, and herpes simplex. It can also be used as a gargle to treat sores and pain in the mouth and throat.

How Is Myrrh Taken?

Because the resin does not dissolve well in water, it is best used as an alcohol extract. The recommended dosage is two to four milliliters of this tincture taken three times daily. See your health-care practitioner for the duration of treatment based upon your specific condition. It is best used in combination with other herbs and is often combined with wild indigo for respiratory tract infections, or with echinacea for other infections. It can also be used topically, as a wash for the treatment of wounds, and as a gargle for the treatment of mouth sores.

Is Myrrh Safe to Use?

Myrrh is very safe. No toxic effects or side effects have been recorded.

Sage

Sage *(Salvia officinalis)* grows wild in southern Europe and in Mediterranean countries. In the United States, it is cultivated as a spice used for cooking. It is an excellent remedy for inflammatory conditions of the mouth and throat.

How Does Sage Work?

Sage contains a high concentration of a volatile oil known as sage oil, which possesses antibacterial activity.

What Is Sage Used to Treat?

The antibacterial action of sage makes it suitable for bacterial infections of the mouth, throat, and tonsils. It is also an excellent remedy for mouth ulcers. In these situations, it is best to use sage as a mouthwash or gargle before swallowing it. Sage can also be used to treat diarrhea, gastritis, and enteritis.

How Is Sage Taken?

It is best to use either an infusion (tea) or a tincture (liquid extract). If used as an infusion, pour a cup of boiling water over two teaspoonfuls of the leaves and leave to infuse for fifteen minutes. This should be drunk three times daily. When using sage to treat mouth infections, gargle with the tea and swish it aroung your mouth before swallowing. If using a tincture, take ten to fifteen drops (two to four milliliters) three times daily. See your health-care practitioner for the duration of treatment based upon your specific condition.

Is Sage Safe to Use?

Long-term and excessive use of sage can cause symptoms of poisoning. Avoid this herb during pregnancy, as it can stimulate contractions of the uterus.

Thyme

Thyme *(Thymus vulgaris)* is another plant that is cultivated for use as a spice for cooking. It is an excellent cough remedy.

Thyme is one of the best antiseptic substances available, which makes it valuable in the treatment of infections.

How Does Thyme Work?

Thyme has a high concentration of volatile oils, which include thymol. This volatile oil is highly antiseptic, which explains why thyme is so valuable in the treatment of infections.

What Is Thyme Used to Treat?

Thyme can be used as an antiseptic for external wounds. Its main use is in the treatment of respiratory infections. It may be used as a gargle to treat tonsillitis, pharyngitis, and laryngitis. It is also an excellent cough remedy, producing expectoration and reducing spasms in the airways, hence, its usefulness in treating bronchitis and asthma.

How Is Thyme Taken?

It is best to use either an infusion (tea) or a tincture (liquid extract). If used as an infusion, pour a cup of boiling water over two teaspoonfuls of the leaves and allow to infuse for fifteen minutes. This should be drunk three times daily. If using a tincture, take ten to fifteen drops (two to four milliliters) three times daily. See your health-care practitioner for the appropriate duration of treatment based upon your specific condition.

Is Thyme Safe to Use?

Thyme is a safe herb to use, even for young children and during pregnancy. Excessive internal use, however, has been shown to cause overstimulation of the thyroid and symptoms of poisoning.

Marigold

Marigold (*Calendula officinalis*), also called calendula, is a flowering garden plant that has also been found to be beneficial in treating infections, especially skin infections. It is an ingredient in many cosmetics, ointments, creams, and soaps.

How Does Marigold Work?

The active chemical constituents of marigold have not yet been identified, but it is known to possess good anti-inflammatory action and to have antifungal activity.

What Is Marigold Used to Treat?

Marigold's main uses are in the treatment of skin conditions, including eczema and dermatitis, as well as wounds, bruises, and skin ulcers. It is ideal for the treatment of minor burns and scalds and for rashes. Because of its antifungal activity, it can be used both externally and internally in the treatment of fungal infections—externally for such conditions as ringworm and athlete's foot, and internally for such conditions as vaginal and intestinal thrush.

How Is Marigold Taken?

It is best to use either an infusion (tea) or a tincture (liquid extract). If used as an infusion, pour a cup of boiling water over two teaspoonfuls of the leaves and allow to infuse for fifteen minutes. This should be drunk three times daily. If using a tincture, take ten to fifteen drops (2–4 ml) three times daily. See your health-care practioner for the appropriate duration of treatment based upon your specific condition. Use a commercial ointment or cream if you wish to apply it externally, and follow the dosage directions on the label.

Is Marigold Safe to Use?

Marigold is a very safe herb to use, even for young children and during pregnancy.

Garlic

Garlic (*Allium sativum*) is well known for its antibiotic properties. It was used by the ancient Egyptians to treat worm infestations and infections, by the Greeks and Romans for tumors, wounds, and generalized infections, and by the Chinese to treat weakness, fatigue, infections, and tumors. In 1858, Louis Pasteur demonstrated the wonderful antibacterial properties of garlic. In both World Wars, garlic saved countless thousands of lives by protecting wounds from becoming infected. When no other antiseptic was available, surface wounds were smeared with crushed garlic and then bandaged.

More recent research has shown that garlic juice can both slow the growth of and kill more than sixty species of fungi and more than twenty species of bacteria, including some of the most virulent. Interestingly, garlic is currently attracting a lot of attention from the medical profession for its ability to lower blood cholesterol, as well as for its anticancer properties.

How Does Garlic Work?

The oil in garlic contains the active substance responsible for its antibiotic/antimicrobial properties. This oil contains a sulfur compound called allicin that kills bacteria and fungi. When eaten, the oil enters the digestive system and is absorbed into the bloodstream. Because of this, garlic is best used for infections of the digestive and respiratory tracts. The herb is excreted via the lungs, hence the strong sulfur-type odor of the breath after garlic has been consumed.

What Is Garlic Used to Treat?

Garlic is most effective in the treatment of respiratory infections, such as influenza, bronchitis, and recurrent colds. It has also been found that garlic supports the development of the beneficial bacteria in the digestive tract, as well as kills intestinal parasites. Garlic is also helpful in the treatment of such intestinal infections as cholera, dysentery, and typhoid.

How Is Garlic Taken?

Eat one clove three times daily. If the smell is problematic, take garlic oil capsules three times daily.

Is Garlic Safe to Use?

Since garlic is a food and not a medicine, it is very safe to use with no known side effects.

Wormwood

Wormwood *(Artemisia absinthum)*, also known as absinthe, grows along roadsides in parts of Canada and in northwestern United States. It is indigenous to Europe. As the name suggests, wormwood is a good remedy for worm infestation, especially of roundworms.

How Does Wormwood Work?

It is thought that its antihelmintic (antiworm) properties are due to certain bitter chemicals in the herb called sesquiterpenes. It is a bitter herb and, therefore, has the effect of stimulating and invigorating the whole digestive system.

What Is Wormwood Used to Treat?

Its main use is as a bitter to stimulate the digestive process. In addition, because of the sesquiterpenes, it is used in the treatment of worm infestations, especially of roundworm and pinworm. The oil can be used topically as a local anesthetic.

How Is Wormwood Taken?

When used as a bitter, it should be taken as an infusion or

tincture. If used as an infusion, pour a cup of boiling water over two teaspoonfuls of the leaves and allow to infuse for fifteen minutes. This should be drunk three times daily. If using a tincture, take ten to fifteen drops (two to four milliliters) three times daily. See your health-care practitioner for the appropriate duration of treatment based upon your specific condition. If using this herb to get rid of worms, commercially prepared tablet forms can be used to avoid the bitter taste. Follow the dosage recommendations on the label.

Is Wormwood Safe to Use?

In large doses, wormwood can cause insomnia, nightmares, vomiting, and convulsions, and so must be used with caution. It may also cause spontaneous abortion during pregnancy, so should not be used by pregnant women. These side effects are due to a constituent of the oil in the herb called thujone. It is, however, possible to get a thujone-free extract of the herb. Wormwood was the basis for the alcoholic drink absinthe, which was popular in the nineteenth century but was subsequently banned because when too much was consumed, side effects were apparent. It is, therefore, best used under the supervision of a qualified health-care practioner.

Thuja

Thuja *(Thuja occidentalis)* is also known as the tree of life, arborvitae, white cedar, and yellow cedar. A woody plant belonging to the Cypress family, it is native to the northeastern part of North America, where it was used mainly as an herbal preparation. It was imported to Europe during the sixteenth century and became well known medicinally as a homeopathic preparation. It is cultivated in Europe in gardens, particularly as hedging.

The positive effects of thuja when applied topically to skin conditions, warts, and genital warts has been described in numerous articles. As far back as 1838, Dr. Warnatz reported that he had used thuja to heal a patient with warts on the penis and scrotum that previously had been unresponsive to treatment.

Good results have been reported by numerous researchers since then. Most of the research relating to thuja centers on the treatment of skin warts and the use of thuja as an external application, rather than as an internal medicine. In 1949, Dr. Halter described the treatment of warts using thuja internally, with no external application at all. It is now believed that thuja has an inhibitory action on viruses. It can, therefore, be taken internally for a whole range of viral diseases of the respiratory tract, such as bronchitis, laryngitis, and sore throats of a viral origin, and viral diseases of the digestive tract.

How Does Thuja Work?

Thuja has been investigated mostly as an antiviral substance. Unequivocal evidence of its strong antiviral properties was presented by a Dr. Khurana in 1971, who investigated the effects of this herb on a host of different viruses. Others have confirmed its antiviral effect, although the active chemicals have not yet been identified. According to some researchers, thuja possesses antibacterial properties as well, so it may be useful in the treatment of infected surface wounds and burns.

Despite the fact that it has been in use for centuries in folk medicine and homeopathy, little scientific research has been done on thuja, compared with the amount of research that has been done on other herbs, such as echinacea.

What Is Thuja Used to Treat?

Thuja is used mainly for the treatment of viral infections. If you have a cold, flu, viral sore throat, viral laryngitis, or viral bronchitis, then it should be taken internally as a homeopathic preparation (see Chapter 6). For viral skin infections, such as warts and genital warts, thuja can be applied directly to the wart. The herb also has a marked antifungal effect and so is useful for external fungal infections, such as ringworm.

Another effect that has been well documented in the scientific literature is the ability of thuja to prevent a common tropical disease called bilharziasis. This is caused by a worm, the larvae of which can penetrate human skin when a person comes in contact with fresh water. When applied to the skin, thuja has been shown to prevent the larvae from penetrating the skin. Thuja has also been reported to counteract the ill effects of smallpox vaccination.

How Is Thuja Taken?

Thuja is best taken internally as a homeopathic preparation (see Chapter 6) or applied externally in the form of a liquid herbal extract. It can also be taken internally as an herbal extract, primarily to treat viral infections of the respiratory tract, but this should only be done under medical supervision. Thuja can also be applied externally to treat skin warts and genital warts, and fungal infections, such as ringworm. See your health-care practitioner for appropriate dosages and duration of treatment based upon your specific condition.

Is Thuja Safe to Use?

When taken internally in high dosages or in lower dosages over a long period of time, herbal preparations of thuja were found to cause severe side effects, such as inducing contractions of the uterus during pregnancy, and symptoms of poisoning. These effects do not occur when thuja is applied topically to the skin or when it is used as a homeopathic preparation. Hence, it is safe to use thuja as a homeopathic preparation but not as an herbal extract. The latter is safe to use on skin lesions only. Thuja is an herb that is best administered by a doctor or qualified herbalist, especially if it is being taken as an oral medicine. Research has shown that if a cold water/alcohol extraction method is used in preparing the herbal medicine, the side effects are absent, making it much safer to take orally.

Echinacea-Baptisia Compound

Echinacea–baptisia compound is an exciting product. It is a blend of the liquid extracts of the root, leaf, and flower of the echinacea plant *(Echinacea purpurea* and *Echinacea angustifolia),* wild indigo root *(Baptisia tinctoria),* thuja leaf *(Thuja occidentalis),* boneset leaf and flower *(Eupatorium perfoliatum),* and prickly ash bark *(Xanthoxylum clava-herculis).* During the last five years, I have seen a particular need for echinacea and wild indigo among my patients, so it is good to be able to use a product that combines the immune-enhancing properties of these herbs with the antiviral properties of thuja.

How Does Echinacea-Baptisia Compound Work?

The herbs that make up echinacea–baptisia compound contain chemicals that work to strengthen the body's immune system. These chemicals stimulate the production of T-lymphocytes and macrophages, the cells in the immune systems are that work to fight disease. In this way, the chemicals activate the immune system, protecting against infection and shortening the duration of existing infection.

What Is Echinacea-Baptisia Compound Used to Treat?

Echinacea-baptisia compound is used by individuals whose immune systems are either weakened or suppressed. It can be used to treat abscesses, asthma, boils, ear infections, hay fever, impetigo, respiratory tract infections, sinusitis, and streptococcal sore throats. It can also be used to enhance one's white blood cell count following anticancer treatment, such as radio- or chemotherapy, and to reduce susceptibility to infection due to lowered resistance.

How Is Echinacea-Baptisia Compound Taken?

Echinacea-baptisia compound is dispensed in a liquid form, and it is recommended that twenty to forty drops be taken two to five times a day to treat acute conditions. For chronic or recurring conditions, the recommended dosage is twenty to forty drops in water, to be taken two or three times a day. Either dosage should be done six days a week for six weeks. After the initial six weeks, no drops should be taken for one full week. If this treatment is not successful, the cycle may be repeated. It may take one to three months of treatment in this manner for the compound's full effects to be felt.

Is Echinacea-Baptisia Compound Safe to Use?

There are no side effects associated with the use of echinacea-baptisia compound. However, as echinacea-baptisia compound contains thuja, which can stimulate the walls of the uterus and cause them to contract, this product is best avoided during pregnancy.

HERBAL MEDICINE AND THE MEDICAL PROFESSION

Why has the medical profession not embraced herbal medicines in the same way it has synthetically produced drugs? I believe the answer has to do with money and power, although teaching methods in medical schools are also a factor.

First of all, there is no big money in herbs. Herbal medicines cannot be patented, so there is no incentive to produce them on a large scale. Drugs, regardless of whether they are produced synthetically or isolated from herbal extracts, can be patented, bottled, and sold for incredible sums of money. This is what pharmaceutical companies do. This is why they are so wealthy and capable of financing so many medical projects.

The curriculum of medical education is another reason that herbal medicine has not been embraced by the medical profession. Medical education is not holistic. Often, it makes no attempt to deal with people on anything other than a physical level. The main form of treatment, even when dealing with sensitive emotional issues, is pharmaceutical drugs. For the most part, no attempt is made to educate doctors in issues as fundamental as nutrition. You only have to look at the food served in hospital cafeterias and coffee shops to see the incredible lack of awareness among doctors in this regard—ironically, it is often their job to treat people with nutritional imbalances.

Herbal medicine and nutrition must form the cornerstone of medical therapeutics if people are to be healed rather than

Natural Alternatives to Antibiotics at Work

Jennifer was 13 years old and had been diagnosed as having glandular fever by her family doctor. This is a viral illness that causes a fever and enlarged, tender lymph glands in the early stages. It may also cause liver and spleen enlargement. Glandular fever is a severe illness, and it can take months for a patient to completely recover from it. Later, it can go on to cause chronic fatigue. Jennifer's blood tests showed that the virus was still active in her body.

Initially, I prescribed two measures to treat Jennifer: an immune booster and high-dose vitamin C therapy, as the vitamin C needs of the body increase considerably during an infection. This resulted in a marked improvement in her symptoms, and she was able to return to school. Within six weeks, her blood tests returned to normal, but she still complained of discomfort in the upper right quadrant of her abdomen. Examination showed that her liver was still enlarged and tender. I gave her milk thistle (*Silybum marianum*), a wonderful herb for assisting liver function. Two months later, Jennifer was fully recovered.

simply treated. At present, the only form of therapeutics taught to medical students in college is pharmacology—the study and use of chemical drugs. The medical profession must choose between money and power on the one hand and the good of humanity on the other. When next you see or hear negative reports in the media about herbal medicine, remember that this is the most important form of medicine for the majority of people on the planet, especially those who cannot afford expensive drugs.

The regard the modern medical establishment holds for herbal medicine is clearly reflected in the attitude of the U.S. National Cancer Institute. On the one hand, the institute issues statements confirming that up to 60 percent of cancers in humans can be prevented through better nutrition and a less stressful lifestyle. This is quite an admission by a body of scientists and doctors who are provided with large sums of money to find cures for these cancers. However, on the other hand, the very same body of people spend approximately one percent of their budget on nutritional research. If this is not revealing enough, the same institute spends vast amounts of money isolating chemicals from herbs that grow in the Amazon River basin of South America.

In Chapter 9, which deals with nutrition, I state that manufacturers of processed foods are interested in profits, not in your health. Unfortunately, it appears that the same can be said of modern medicine and pharmaceutics. Huge sums of money are being spent on isolating chemicals from herbs that are known to have anticancer properties. These chemicals are then mass produced, packaged, and sold for enormous profits. Using the natural herb is safer and healthier. If the natural herb is used alongside nutritional medicine and changes in lifestyle, patients can participate in their own care and use fewer potentially harmful substances to heal their bodies.

When I was in medical school, I learned ways to suppress the immune system with drugs such as steroids, azathioprine, and cyclosporin, which are used in transplant patients and in the treatment of certain autoimmune diseases. I did not learn how to enhance immunity. It was only years later that I discovered that there are, in fact, ways to boost people's immunity.

It is encouraging to see herbs such as echinacea, wild indigo, and thuja being used more commonly by patients to protect themselves and their families. Encourage your family physician to learn more about these herbs so that your doctor may prescribe them for you too. Because of the high level of safety associated with echinacea and wild indigo, you may use them without a prescription. If in doubt, consult a medical herbalist, pharmacist, or doctor trained in natural medicine.

CHAPTER 6

HOMEOPATHIC MEDICINE

Small Is Beautiful

Homeopathy is a system of healing based on the use of very small amounts of substances, which in larger doses would cause illness in a healthy person, to treat illness. For the most part, homeopathic medicines are derived from herbs. A few are also derived from minerals, such as sulfur and phosphorus. Minute doses of these herbs and minerals are used to stimulate the healing powers of the body in a very specific way. For example, if you have a cough, a homeopath will use a remedy to stimulate the cough, explaining that the cough is the body's way of expelling an irritant, such as a virus, inhaled dust, or smoke. In other words, homeopathic medicines stimulate the body's natural drive to restore itself to health in order to heal the patient. Echinacea and wild indigo, herbs you have already read about, are often used in homeopathic form to stimulate the body's defenses when an infection is present in the body.

Simply explained, homeopathic medicines enhance your own natural healing powers. They are very safe, even in newborn babies, as they have no side effects. Much like conventional medicines, they come in many different forms, including tablets, drops, ampules, suppositories, and nasal sprays.

Drops are the easiest form of homeopathic remedies to take, especially for children. If an acute condition is being treated, one should take ten drops every hour or even half hour, for most remedies. This dosage should be reduced to three times daily once improvement in symptoms is noticed. You may stop taking the drops when symptoms are gone. For chronic conditions, take ten drops three times daily until symptoms disappear. These dosages are for adults and children over the age of twelve. Children between the ages of six and twelve should take five drops three times daily and children younger than six should take three to four drops three times daily. If the medicine comes in an ampule for injection, it is best to seek dosage recommendations from a health-care practitioner.

Homeopathic remedies are small doses of mainly plant and mineral substances that have undergone a process of dilution with water and of being vigorously shaken (succussion). This process of dilution and succussion is called potentization. A solution may consist of one part homeopathic substance diluted in nine parts of water (a 1:10 dilution) or one part substance in ninety-nine parts water (a 1:100 dilution). It is then vigorously shaken to activate the solution.

Potentization can be repeated many times and determines the potency of the solution. If a solution was potentized six times, it is given a potency of 6. If a substance was potentized in a 1 in 10 dilution, this is represented by the Roman numeral X. If a substance was potentized in a 1 in 100 dilution, it is represented by the Roman numeral C. For example, if echinacea was potentized in a 1 in 10 dilution six times, it is called Echinacea 6X.

There are two forms of homeopathy currently being practiced in the United States and Europe—simple and complex homeopathy. All simple and many complex homeopathic remedies are available at health-food stores.

SIMPLE HOMEOPATHY

Simple homeopathy is the classical or more traditional form of homeopathy. This type of homeopathy is based on the use of only one remedy at any one time—that is, only a single remedy used in a single potency is used to treat a single illness. A practitioner of simple homeopathy will select a remedy on the basis of a detailed history from the patient—the homeopath must try to match the patient's symptoms with a particular remedy. Many of these remedies consist of natural substances that are quite common and familiar to many. For example, chamomilla is the remedy of choice for teething in young children, and belladonna is the remedy of choice for scarlet fever.

Although simple remedies can be slow to work, they are very effective. The choice of remedy for a patient depends very much upon the symptoms exhibited by the patient, as the situations outlined in Tables 6.1 and 6.2 illustrate.

COMPLEX HOMEOPATHY

Complex homeopathy is a newer approach and involves the use of more than one remedy at a time. The majority of homeopathic doctors today practice complex homeopathy, primarily

Table 6.1. Simple Homeopathic Remedies for Tonsillitis

Problem/Symptom	Possible Remedy
Swallowing worsens the sore throat.	Lachesis
Swallowing improves the sore throat.	Ignatia
Symptoms have been suppressed by antibiotics.	Thuja
Only the right side of the throat is involved.	Lycopodium
Tonsils are swollen and/or inflamed.	*Apis mellifica*

Table 6.2. Simple Homeopathic Remedies for Earache

Problem/Symptom	Possible Remedy
The earache follows a cold or measles.	Pulsatilla
There is a yellow discharge from the ear.	Pulsatilla
The earache is worse at night.	Pulsatilla
The child is irritable and does not want to be held.	Chamomilla
The earache is worse upon bending down.	Chamomilla
The child is in severe pain.	Belladonna
The pain spreads into the neck or face.	Belladonna

because it works more rapidly. Complex homeopathy is used to treat acute infections. It is also used to boost one's defenses, to undo the damage that drugs like antibiotics can do to the body, and to detoxify the body.

I prescribe a number of complex homeopathic remedies in my practice. For children with recurrent infections, I prescribe *Echinacea compositum.*

Table 6.3 helps explain the difference between simple and complex remedies. In it, there are examples of one simple and two complex homeopathic remedies. The simple remedy contains one substance, in one strength or potency. The first complex remedy contains one substance in different strengths. The second contains several different substances.

Table 6.3. Simple vs. Complex Homeopathic Remedies

Simple	Echinacea 10X	
Complex	Echinacea 10X	Echinacea 10X
	Echinacea 30X	Baptisia 10X
	Echinacea 100X	Byronia 30X

Echinacea Compositum

A complex remedy that I use frequently is called *Echinacea compositum*, a familiar medicine to a number of my patients. It has a broad spectrum of action. It contains several herbs and other substances, including:

- Echinacea—an immune booster.
- Wild indigo—the remedy of choice in respiratory tract and localized infections, such as sinusitis.
- Bryonia—for congestive symptoms of the mucosa.
- Eupatorium—a decongestant.
- Ipecacuanha—an expectorant, useful if treating a cough.
- Lachesis (snake venom)—an excellent remedy for diseases of the bloodstream.
- Thuja (tree of life)—an antiviral agent, important when an infection has been treated with antibiotics.
- Pokeroot (*Phytolacca americana*)—to drain enlarged lymph glands.
- Cleavers—clears the lymph glands of infection.
- Vaccines against the bacteria *Streptococcus spp.* and *Staphylococcus spp.*
- An anti-flu vaccine.

Echinacea compositum contains lachesis, thuja, pokeroot, and cleavers. It also contains vaccines to treat streptococcal, staphylococcal, and influenza-type infections. It is essential for any doctor who is serious about treating infections safely.

An ampule of *Echinacea compositum* can be taken twice daily until the symptoms of the infection abate, and then once daily for up to ten days. Since the herbal form of echinacea can have a strong taste in the mouth, I often use the homeopathic form for young children. Echinacea compositum is available only in ampules and by prescription. It is not available over the counter. Your health-care practitioner will advise you regarding the dosage, as this will vary depending on the clinical condition.

Engystol

Engystol is another complex remedy often used in combination with echinacea to treat viral infections. It is sold in tablet form and in ampules. It is effective in the treatment of viral infections, such as influenza, the common cold, glandular fever, viral gastroenteritis, herpes simplex infections, and shingles, among others. It is currently being researched as a possible additional treatment for patients with hepatitis and AIDS.

In viral tonsillitis in a child, for example, I would prescribe engystol as an antiviral measure and *Echinacea compositum* to assist the body's defenses. This is a very effective way to overcome an acute infection quickly. I would then continue the drops for seven days to assist the body's recovery. I may use cleavers in herbal or homeopathic form to drain the lymph glands.

UNDOING THE HARM CAUSED BY ANTIBIOTICS

Sometimes it is necessary to treat patients for the adverse effects of antibiotics. There are homeopathic medicines specifically designed to undo the harm that certain antibiotics cause within the body. These homeopathic medicines may even have the same name as the antibiotic, as with the homeopathic remedy tetracycline. When patients see this name, they get confused and can be anxious that I, too, am giving them antibiotics. A

Natural Alternatives to Antibiotics at Work

Unlike so many of my patients, Jackie came to me as the first port of call, not the last. She was suffering from tonsillitis. On examination, her tonsils were inflamed, but there were no white dots on her tonsils, which would have indicated that there was pus present. She also had enlarged lymph glands and a low-grade temperature. I diagnosed viral tonsillitis and prescribed vitamin C, Echinacea compositum ampules, and Engystol for five days. After forty-eight hours of treatment, there was a marked improvement in Jackie's condition. Later, I used cleavers, an herbal medicine, to drain the lymph nodes.

Jackie's case was relatively uncomplicated, and it illustrates just how easy it can be to treat an acute infection using natural medicines. Unfortunately, many of my patients' problems are much more complicated than this, and they sometimes do not respond to such simple measures.

simple explanation, or showing them a page in my homeopathic *Materia Medica* (a book containing a list of homeopathic medicines and what they do), alleviates their anxiety.

Some of the more common adverse effects of antibiotic usage that I've seen in my practice include:

- Abdominal pain or discomfort.
- Alteration of bacterial flora.
- Altered mood.
- Chronic cough.
- A decrease in the blood levels of certain minerals (including zinc, calcium, and magnesium).

- A decrease in the blood levels of certain vitamins (including K, B_2, and B_3).
- Earache.
- Fatigue.
- Impaired immune response.
- Increased flatulence.
- Increased mucus production.
- Itchy ears.
- Nasal congestion.
- Pancreatic damage.
- A sickly feeling in the stomach.

If I see any of these symptoms in a patient, it is a warning to me that antibiotic damage may be present and that a homeopathic "antidote" may be needed at some stage in the course of treatment.

I remember, in particular, a young man who had been on two separate courses of tetracycline for teenage acne. The first course was for a period of six months, followed eight weeks later by a longer course of twelve months. When a broad-spectrum antibiotic has been used for long periods like this, damage is almost inevitable, especially to the digestive system.

I sent this patient for testing and the results showed both pancreatic damage and alterations of the bacterial flora. Testing also indicated the need to use tetracycline in homeopathic form, which I did. This did not solve his acne problem, but it had to be done if this patient was going to show any positive response to medicines meant specifically for his acne.

Such are the difficulties involved with practicing homeopathy. One must first use detoxification remedies to boost the patient's level of health, so that when one prescribes a remedy for a particular complaint, it will be much more likely to have a beneficial effect.

Some patients are so toxic that I could spend weeks or months boosting their level of health prior to treating their symptoms. Their high level of toxicity may be due to a number of factors—drinking tap water that contains heavy metals and chemicals, such as chlorine and fluoride; eating foods with chemical additives; breathing polluted air; using drugs, especially steroids, anti-inflammatory drugs, and antibiotics; stressing the body by working long hours; or by taking stimulants such as tea and coffee.

USING HOMEOPATHY TO CONTROL EPIDEMICS

During the mid-1970s, an epidemic of bacterial meningitis broke out in Brazil. In an attempt to control the spread of the disease, homeopathic doctors inoculated over 18,000 children with a homeopathic vaccine that included the bacteria that cause meningitis *(Neisseria meningitidis)*. This group of children subsequently had a very low incidence of meningitis when compared with other children in the area. The outcome of this treatment clearly shows the importance of homeopath-

Natural Alternatives to Antibiotics at Work

Karen was only 5 years old when her mother brought her to me. The little girl was complaining of recurrent chest infections, tiredness, aches, and pains. Examination of the child and a chest X-ray revealed an infection in the lower right lung. I treated this homeopathically, and the child responded well.

However, two recurrences in the next two months suggested that there was more going on. I was suspicious that the child's immunity was impaired, so I sent her for electronic testing. This revealed that mercury from the mother's dental fillings had affected the child when she was in her mother's womb. A homeopathic detoxification medicine—Metex—specifically designed to remove metals such as mercury from the body was prescribed. Now, one year later, there have been no recurrences of the chest infection.

This case is interesting in two ways. First, it has taught me to ask about the mother's health during pregnancy and about medications taken, and to find out all that I can from her about any sort of activity that may have affected her unborn baby. Second, I have learned to dig deeper when looking for the cause of an ailment, especially if a child fails to get better. I have found electronic testing very helpful in this regard, as it can pick up problems that I would have great difficulty detecting using ordinary clinical methods.

Since testing Karen over eighteen months ago, I have discovered a number of other cases of children who were affected by mercury poisoning from their mother's fillings in utero. Mercury is highly toxic and can leak out of fillings into the mouth. Once swallowed, it is absorbed into the bloodstream. In this way, it can cross the placenta and affect the health of the fetus.

ic medicine and illustrates the need for governments to accept it as a valid form of medicine.

Homeopathic medicine became very popular in Europe and North America because of its success in controlling the cholera epidemics that ravaged these continents during the nineteenth century. Statistics from hospitals in different parts of Europe at the time showed that the death rate in homeopathic hospitals was very low compared with those in conventional hospitals. For example, in 1831 in Raab, Hungary, only six out of 154 homeopathically treated patients died (less than 4 percent), compared with 59 percent of those treated conventionally. Elsewhere in Europe, the mortality rate varied between 2 percent and 20 percent for those treated homeopathically, compared with 50 to 60 percent for those treated conventionally. These statistics, which were suppressed by the governments of these countries so as not to discredit conventional medicine, undoubtedly attest to the power of homeopathy.

More recently, Gaucher et al. (1992) found homeopathic medicines to be so effective in treating a cholera epidemic in Peru that they have now begun a large-scale clinical trial.

I believe that a broad approach to the patient is necessary, involving changes in diet and lifestyle and mineral and vitamin supplementation (where appropriate). I also believe that a quicker acting complex remedy, especially in the case of a streptococcal infection of the tonsils, yields much better results. That is why I prefer to use medicines that are specifically anti-infective. These include *Echinacea compositum* and the herbs you read about earlier.

Homeopathic medicines form the majority of my own prescriptions for patients. I find them extremely effective at treating not just acute infections, but also chronic infections and recurrent infections. I have mentioned only a few to illustrate how they work. There are, in fact, many other preparations on the market today. Homeopathic medicines are cheap, effective, and easy to use. It makes sense to use them in terms of both economics and human health. Remember, however, that it is important to use medicines from reputable companies if you want to benefit from this form of medicine.

CHAPTER 7

NUTRITIONAL SUPPLEMENTATION

Supplementation Is Now the Order of the Day

There are six important nutrients that you need to keep your body healthy—carbohydrates, proteins, fats, vitamins, minerals, and water. Carbohydrates, protein, fat, and water are termed macronutrients because they are needed by the body in large quantities and form the bulk of the diet. Vitamins and minerals are termed micronutrients, as one needs only relatively small amounts of them on a daily basis. Vitamins and minerals are essential for growth, vitality, and well-being. They can also enhance our immunity, improving our resistance to infection and reducing the need for drugs. Save for a few exceptions, vitamins and minerals cannot be manufactured by your body. Therefore, we must obtain them from food or supplements.

DO YOU NEED VITAMIN AND MINERAL SUPPLEMENTS?

There is much debate about this issue among scientists, doctors, nutritionists, and patients. It is best, as it is with any controversial issue, to study the arguments and then adopt a common-sense approach.

The Medical and Scientific Argument

Most doctors and scientists would argue that supplementation with vitamins and minerals for most patients is unnecessary. They would argue, as I did for some time, that a well-
balanced diet, containing lots of fresh fruits and vegetables
and whole foods would provide sufficient micronutrients.
Most doctors would also argue that the Recommended Daily
Allowances (RDA), the guidelines for daily nutrient intake
set down by a group of government scientists, are adequate
for good health. Having been trained as a scientist and a doctor, I understand this argument and agreed with it for many
years. In the last ten years, however, I have read much and
have attended many seminars on nutritional medicine and
have come to realize that this argument does not hold water
anymore.

The Alternative Health Care Argument

Many professionals working in the field of natural medicine
would argue that vitamin and mineral supplementation is
absolutely essential. They base this argument on several
important facts. First, much of the American diet consists of
processed foods, which are devoid of many essential
micronutrients, and many of our plant foods are grown in
soils that are depleted of nutrients, which prohibits the plants
from soaking up these nutrients. Because of the economic
pressure put on fruit and vegetable growers to supply the
steady demand for produce, the soil is not given time to recu-
perate between plantings, but rather must sustain one crop
after the next, and so on. Because many of these crops are
sprayed with pesticides, these chemicals enter the soil and
damage it further.

Further, the RDAs, on which medical doctors base the
amount of nutrients that a person needs, were created to prevent deficiencies. They are insufficient to maintain optimal
health. One needs high levels of vitamins and minerals on a

daily basis to ensure efficient functioning of the body. In fact, most medical doctors and scientists have little or no training in nutritional medicine, and so are often quite ignorant about the subject. Recently, my son David was in the hospital. In the bed next to him was a 9 year-old girl whose mother was very knowledgeable about natural medicine. The surgeon who operated on her daughter entered the room as she and I were having a discussion about monosodium glutamate (MSG), a flavor enhancer added to many foods that has many effects on the body. She asked the surgeon what he thought about MSG, and his reply was, "What is MSG? I've never heard of it." So when consulting a professional about nutrient supplementation, first be sure the person is well learned in the subject, as you may know more about it than he or she does.

HOW VITAMINS AND MINERALS WORK

The macronutrients, especially carbohydrates, provide your body with energy. To release this energy, micronutrients are needed. If you imagine that your body is the internal combustion energy of a car—the macronutrients represent the fuel, and the micronutrients are the spark plugs—then you will begin to get an idea of how vitamins and minerals actually work in the body. Micronutrients are vital for numerous chemical or enzyme reactions that control metabolism. For example, zinc is essential in over 200 enzyme reactions in the body. Hence, a deficiency in zinc can have wide-ranging effects. Now you can understand how a deficiency in a single vitamin or mineral can endanger your health.

Vitamins and minerals regulate the conversion of food into energy in the body. Most of the food we eat is broken down in the small intestine and then absorbed into the bloodstream. It is then transported in the portal vein to the liver, where it is broken down further to release energy. In the process of converting food into energy, harmful free radicals are produced, and if they are not eliminated, they can set the stage for degenerative diseases, such as heart disease, arthritis, premature aging, and cancer.

In the release of energy from the foods we eat, the B vitamins and magnesium play a vital role; these micronutrients work together as a team, the presence of one enhancing the function of another. Other micronutrients act to protect the body from the potential damage of the free radicals. Vitamins A, C, and E, as well as the minerals selenium, zinc, and manganese, play important roles in damage limitation, so preventing the onset of degenerative diseases. These micronutrients also work together as a team, enhancing each other's effects.

This may give you some insight into the way in which micronutrients work. Remember how important it is to take vitamins and minerals together and never in isolation, with few exceptions; so, if using a supplement, be sure that it has a number of both vitamins and minerals together, as this is how they work in the body.

BUYING AND STORING YOUR VITAMIN AND MINERAL SUPPLEMENTS

Most micronutrients are extracted from plant and animal sources, although many vitamins can now be made synthetically. The source is usually stated on the container. Micronutrient supplements are found most often in tablet or capsule form, but they are also sold as powders. Tablets are the most convenient forms and have longer shelf lives than do powders. Capsules are used for the fat-soluble vitamins A, D, and E. Powders have the advantage of having no fillers, binders, or other additives, but are less convenient.

Vitamin and mineral supplements should be stored in a cool, dry place, away from direct sunlight and in a well-closed container. If this is done, unopened supplements should last for two to three years. Once opened, they should last up to twelve months.

TAKING YOUR VITAMIN AND MINERAL SUPPLEMENTS

The best time for taking supplements is after meals. They are derived from food and so should be taken with food for maximum absorption. The water-soluble vitamins do not stay in the body for long. They are not stored by the body, remaining only for about two to four hours. They are absorbed into the bloodstream, and any vitamins that are not utilized are quickly excreted. The fat-soluble vitamins are stored in fat tissue and the liver, and can remain in the body for up to twenty-four hours. Because some of the micronutrients are excreted quite rapidly from the body, it is best to take some after each meal, rather than all at once. If taking them after each meal is inconvenient, then take half the daily dosage after breakfast and the other half after dinner.

Dosages depend on the patient and any clinical conditions that may be present. Recommended dosages will also vary from practitioner to practitioner, depending on their backgrounds and opinions. The table on page 110 shows some supplements and the dosages that I recommend to maintain optimum health; however, the final decision must rest with your health-care practitioner, who knows your health limitations. The following recommended dosages are for adults and children weighing 100 pounds or more. Dosages for smaller children will vary according to the age and weight of the child. Generally, children six years of age and older and under 70 pounds can be given half the adult dose. Those between 70 and 100 pounds can be given three-quarters of the adult dose. A child under the age of six should take formulations specifically designed for young children.

A realistic option would be to buy food that has been organically grown, and to take nutritional supplements to help make up for what is missing in your diet. If you do decide to take a nutritional supplement, there are many for you to choose from. In the text that follows, you will find dis-

Table 7.1 Immune-Enhancing Vitamins and Minerals

Nutrient	Daily Dosages
Vitamin A	10,000 IU
Beta-carotene	15,000 IU
Vitamin B_1	50 mg
Vitamin B_2	50 mg
Vitamin B_3	50–100 mg
Vitamin B_5	50 mg
Vitamin B_6	50 mg
Vitamin B_{12}	300 mcg
Biotin	300 mcg
Choline	100 mg
Folic acid	800 mcg
Inositol	100 mg
Para-aminobenzoic acid	50 mg
Vitamin C	1,000–3,000 mg
Vitamin D	400–800 IU
Vitamin E	400–800 IU
Bioflavonoids	500 mg
Calcium	1,500 mg
Iron	20 mg
Magnesium	750 mg
Manganese	10 mg
Selenium	200 mcg
Zinc	50 mg

cussion of those nutritional supplements that I feel are the most important and the most useful in the prevention of infections.

VITAMIN A

Vitamin A is very helpful in enhancing immunity. It plays an important role in maintaining the integrity of all the epithelial surfaces in the body, i.e. the skin, as well as the lining of the respiratory and digestive tracts. These surfaces are exposed to the external environment and form the first line of defense against foreign invaders. Vitamin A also stimulates numerous immunity processes, such as antibody production. It is also an antioxidant. For these reasons, vitamin A is very effective in protecting the body from infection.

Vitamin A is a fat-soluble vitamin, and so requires fats as well as minerals to be properly absorbed from the digestive system. It occurs in nature as vitamin A and as provitamin A (known as carotenes), which is converted in the liver into vitamin A. The carotenes are plant pigments that protect the plant from being damaged during photosynthesis by acting as powerful antioxidants. The best known of the carotenes is beta-carotene. Beta-carotene appears to work in a similar way in the body as it does in plants, by neutralizing free radicals and so preventing them from causing damage.

Vitamin A is found naturally in animal sources, such as liver, fish liver oil, eggs, and dairy products. Beta-carotene can be found in dark green and yellow-orange fruits and vegetables, such as carrots, broccoli, peppers, apricots, and papayas.

Dosages over 100,000 IU daily can produce symptoms of toxicity in adults if taken for several months. Dosages over 10,000 IU can cause toxicity in young children. Signs of toxicity include skin rashes, small cracks and scales on the lips and at the corners of the mouth, nausea, vomiting, diarrhea, blurred vision, fatigue, headache, and liver enlargement. Those with any form of liver disease should not take more than 10,000 IU daily from all sources.

VITAMIN B₆ (PYRIDOXINE)

Pyridoxine is involved in a wide range of bodily functions, including activating many enzyme systems in the body, assisting the absorption of vitamin B_{12}, and aiding immune system function. A deficiency of vitamin B_6 causes a decrease in the number and activiy of lymphocytes, a type of white blood cell, and a decrease in antibody production. In other words, a vitamin B_6 deficiency leads to depressed immunity. Those who consume an excessive amount of protein, who abuse alcohol, who are receiving estrogen therapy, or who take oral contraceptives, antidepressants, or diuretics are probably deficient in vitamin B_6.

Vitamin B_6 is found naturally in brewer's yeast, wheat bran, wheat germ, carrots, chicken, eggs, fish, and meat. In supplement form, it is best taken as part of a B complex formula that contains at least 50 milligrams of vitamin B_6.

Daily doses of more than 2,000 milligrams can cause neurological disorders, such as night restlessness, as well as dependency. Do not take more than 500 milligrams per day. Vitamin B_6 supplementation can reduce a diabetic's need for extra insulin, increasing the risk for hypoglycemia (low blood sugar levels) if one continues taking the regular dose of insulin. Anyone taking the Parkinson's disease drug levodopa should not take vitamin B_6 supplements, as they interact adversely with each other.

VITAMIN C

Vitamin C was the nutrient that first stirred my interest in nutritional medicine. In the early 1970s, I was studying at Trinity College in Dublin. At that time, the pathology department was looking at the effect of viral infections on the levels of vitamin C in white blood cells. Students with colds were paid a nominal amount—the equivalent of one dollar and fifty cents—to give blood samples for analysis. The results of the study confirmed the findings of other researchers, namely that vitamin C is important for the proper functioning of white blood cells.

Dr. Linus Pauling, the Nobel Prize laureate, had been preaching the benefits of vitamin C for years. He himself took large doses of it daily. His research, as well as that of others, showed that people taking 200 to 1,000 milligrams of vitamin C daily had fewer colds than those who were given a placebo (an inactive tablet).

In 1965, the American biochemist Irwin Stone conducted research into the biochemical effects of vitamin C in the body. On the basis of his findings, he proposed that for the maintenance of good health, the optimum daily intake of vitamin C should be 1,000 to 5,000 milligrams.

Both Dr. Pauling and Dr. Stone found it interesting that the American Academy of Sciences recommended a daily vitamin C intake of only 60 milligrams for humans, but for laboratory monkeys, they recommended 2,000 milligrams per day. In addition, it is known that a gorilla in the wild obtains up to 5,000 milligrams of vitamin C per day in its diet. Clearly, we humans need much higher levels of vitamin C than are being recommended at present.

Dr. Robert Cathcart, the orthopedic surgeon renowned for designing the artificial hip, has also turned to nutritional medicine—he prescribes massive doses of vitamin C to patients with infections. The results are quite remarkable. He has shown that it is possible to successfully treat an infection using nothing but high-dose vitamin C therapy. According to F.R. Klenner in "Virus Pneumonia and Its Treatment With Vitamin C" (*Journal of Southern Medicine and Surgery* 2, 1948), even viral pneumonia can be treated successfully using high-dose vitamin C therapy alone. However, for serious infection, vitamin C must be administered intravenously by a physician.

Vitamin C is essential for the activity of white blood cells. White blood cells are like soldiers in the body—they fight off invading pathogens, such as viruses, bacteria, or fungi. When there are high levels of vitamin C in the body, these white blood cells become much more active. Their ability to defend the body against harmful bacteria is enhanced.

Various research projects have addressed the role of vitamin C in increasing the levels of interferon, an antiviral substance produced in the body. This increases the level of antibody in the bloodstream and boosts the activity of the thymus gland, a gland that has a very important role in the immune system. Many doctors and researchers use very high doses of vitamin C in the treatment of AIDS, cancer, and other diseases in which boosting the immune function is of primary importance.

Vitamin C has a positive effect on different parts of the immune system, making it easier for the body to deal with infection. Studies have also shown that taking vitamin C in large doses prevents an infection from developing in the first place, shortens the duration of an infection, and reduces the severity of the disease. In 1977, Dr. J. Asfora conducted one such study on the effects of vitamin C therapy in cold treatment. He gave 1,000 milligrams of vitamin C or a placebo to a group of doctors and patients who had colds. Some took the pills on the first day of the cold, others on the second day, and others on the third day of their cold. Those taking vitamin C experienced fewer symptoms and developed fewer complications. Dr. Pauling explains that vitamin C is necessary for white blood cells to destroy invading viruses or bacteria. When high levels of vitamin C are present, white blood cells fight viruses and bacteria more effectively; when there are low levels of vitamin C in the body, this ability is reduced.

Despite all of the evidence that vitamin C is beneficial to the treatment of so many maladies, the medical profession continues to overlook its use as a valid method of treatment. The underuse of vitamin C is one example of the prevailing attitude within the medical profession that nutrition is of little consequence to health. However, there is a ray of hope that ideas and beliefs may be changing. The effectiveness of vitamin C in cancer treatment was the subject of a 1991 con-

Nutritional Supplements at Work

One example of the life-and-death importance of vitamin C may be found in Dr. Kalokerinos' book *Every Second Child*. In the 1960s, while working in rural Australia, Dr. Kalokerinos observed that many Aboriginal children and some European children died suddenly even though they had only minor symptoms, such as a runny nose and a mild cough. He postulated that these children, who died from what was believed to be (but not yet termed at that time) Sudden Infant Death Syndrome (SIDS), were actually suffering from vitamin C deficiency. The basis for this hypothesis was his clinical experience—when these children were dying and not responding to antibiotics or other life-saving drugs, an injection of vitamin C led to very dramatic and instant recovery. This happened so many times that he soon realized that these children were suffering from scurvy. The medical profession in Australia treated his work with disbelief. Remember that most doctors are not taught about the clinical use of vitamins and minerals in medical school.

Dr. Kalokerinos also noticed that when normal childhood vaccines—tuberculosis, polio, diphtheria, pertussis, and tetanus—were given to Aboriginal children, 50 percent of the children died. He believed that these children had a low immunity as a result of a poor diet—they lived on processed food, white sugar, white bread, and ate little or no fresh fruits or vegetables. Dr. Kalokerinos then started giving each child vitamin C in a dose of 100 mg per day for three days (the day prior to vaccination, the day of vaccination, and the day following) for each month of age—a 3-month-old child received 300 mg daily, a 4-month-old child received 400 mg daily, and so on. When they were later immunized, none of these children died. Because this work has been validated by many others, a number of doctors in different parts of the world now use similar doses of vitamin C around the time of vaccination.

If you are a parent, vitamin C can be helpful to you. Using vitamin C, you can protect your child from the potentially damaging effects of vaccination, particularly the measles-mumps-rubella vaccine, which is surrounded by a great deal of controversy. Use the above dosage of vitamin C on the day before, the day of, and the day following vaccination. This applies to any vaccine given in the first two years of life. For children over the age of two years, especially with the measles-mumps-rubella vaccine, administer the dosage for seven days instead of three.

ference organized by the National Cancer Institute of America. This conference was helpful in informing both doctors and patients of the benefits of taking vitamin C on a daily basis. According to Dr. Gladys Block, an epidemiologist in the Division of Cancer Prevention and Control at the Natural Cancer Institute, vitamin C has been shown to be protective against cancer of the lung, larynx, colorectal tract, esophagus, stomach, pancreas, bladder, cervix, endometrium, and breast, as well as childhood brain tumors. These findings seem to represent a change of heart within the medical profession—recognition that perhaps nutritional medicine has something important to add to medical science, something that doctors can no longer afford to ignore.

Daily requirements for vitamin C vary considerably, not only among individuals, but also within the same individual from day to day. For example, when you are healthy and feeling well, your daily requirement may be as low as 200 milligrams. But if you become stressed for any reason, your daily requirement may rise to 1,000 milligrams. In addition, if you are in the early stages of developing an infection, your daily requirement may be even higher. In the treatment of an acute infection, I recommend that adults take 10,000 milligrams of vitamin C for two days, then 5,000 milligrams of vitamin C daily for two days, then 2,000 to 3,000 milligrams as a daily maintenance dose for one week. Children between the ages of six and twelve should take half of this recommended dose. For children under the age of six consult your health-care practitioner for recommended dosages. Since this vitamin is not stored in the body, there is no concern of overloading the body with too much of it.

The body's requirements for vitamin C also increases in the case of pregnancy, surgery, and trauma. On average, however, the daily vitamin C requirement has been estimated, biochemically, as being between 1,000 milligrams and 5,000 milligrams. As a general guideline, I suggest that my adult patients take 1,000 to 2,000 milligrams of vitamin C as a preventative measure. Children should take doses that are slightly lower based upon their age and weight.

Vitamin C is available as ascorbic acid alone or combined with minerals (called mineral ascorbates). If you are taking large amounts of vitamin C it is best to take the ascorbic acid, as it is more readily absorbed into the bloodstream. However, pure ascorbic acid has quite a low pH, and this acid can cause irritation to the stomach in those who have low levels of hydrochloric acid in their stomachs, such as the elderly. If the ascorbic acid is irritating to your stomach, the mineral ascorbates (such as calcium ascorbate, magnesium ascorbate, and sodium ascorbate) can be taken instead. These are nonacidic and less irritating to the stomach.

If taking doses greater than 1,000 milligrams per day, it is easier to take vitamin C in powdered form. For smaller doses and children's doses, the commercial tablets available in most pharmacies are perfectly fine.

Since vitamin C is a water-soluble vitamin, there is little risk of toxicity associated with its use. At the talks and seminars that I give, I am often asked about the risk of developing kidney stones as a result of taking very high doses of vitamin C. Research in this area (Hoffer, 1985) indicates that, in the majority of people, there is very little risk of this happening. In fact, it is only those individuals who have family histories of kidney stone development who need to take care. To further minimize this risk, it is recommended that susceptible individuals take 500 milligrams of magnesium daily and 50 milligrams of pyridoxine (vitamin B_6) twice daily.

ZINC

Zinc is a trace mineral (a mineral required in small amounts) that is necessary for your health. Unfortunately, zinc deficiency is one of the most common micronutrient deficiencies. Even mild zinc deficiency can have enormous repercussions on a person's health. This is because this trace mineral is required by more than 200 hundred enzymes for their activity. In fact, many chemical reactions in the body need zinc. A zinc deficiency can affect a wide number of important reactions in the body. Signs of zinc deficiency include growth retardation, poor appetite, mental lethargy, underfunctioning of the sex glands, and increased susceptibility to infections. If your child has a poor appetite, suspect a zinc deficiency.

Zinc is now firmly established as a major protector of the immune system and an important disease fighter. It has been clearly established that zinc is essential for immune system function carried out by the white blood cells. Acrodermatitis enteropathica is a rare disorder that causes its victims to be more susceptible to infections and die young. These patients have defects in the activity of their white blood cells, as well as in other parts of their immune system. This condition is treatable with zinc.

Research has shown a definite decrease in the number of circulating T-lymphocytes, which fight infection, in patients who are over the age of 70. This is one of the groups most at risk of recurrent infections. It is now being suggested that one of the reasons that the immune system becomes weaker with age may be because zinc levels are lower at this time of life. Other studies have shown that patients with AIDS have significantly lower blood levels of zinc when compared with a control group. This suggests a role for zinc supplementation in these patients.

The RDA for zinc is 15 milligrams daily for adults and 10 milligrams for children. I, however, recommend a minimum daily intake of 10 to 15 milligrams in children, and 20 to 30 milligrams for adults, especially where there is a history of recurrent infections. This is more than the Recommended Daily Allowances (RDAs), but it is necessary if one is to correct the deficiency quickly and reduce the incidence of infection.

You can also supplement your daily intake of zinc by adding certain foods to your diet. The best dietary sources of zinc are whole grain cereals, legumes, and meats. Oysters also have very high levels of zinc. I normally recommend zinc supplementation for a three-month period. After this time, I assess the patient's health and make recommendations based on his or her status.

Certain foods can affect the way that your body is able to absorb and use zinc. Fiber, iron, and calcium diminish the amount of zinc that you are able to absorb. Excessively high amounts of fiber in the diet can reduce the absorption of zinc across the bowel wall into the bloodstream.

There are no adverse effects associated with low-dose zinc supplementation. Large doses of zinc, however—doses around 300 milligrams daily—may have a negative effect on the immune system. For this reason, correct dosage is important. In one particular study, eleven men took 150 milligrams of zinc twice a day for six weeks. This resulted in a significant reduction in their immune function (Chandra, 1984). I recommend that you take no more than 50 milligrams per day. Because zinc competes with copper for absorption across the bowel wall, high doses of zinc could create a deficiency of copper. If you are taking a high-dose zinc supplement that contains more zinc than the doses I have suggested above, it would be wise to include some copper in your supplementation schedule. A dose of copper that is one-tenth of the zinc dosage should be sufficient. In other words, if you are taking 50 milligrams of zinc daily, you should also take 5 milligrams of copper.

Unfortunately, the food that is available to us has become nutrient-poor because of imperfect production practices. As a result of this, we may sometimes find ourselves lacking, or deficient, in nutrients that our bodies need. These deficiencies can cause adverse effects within our bodies, including causing us to be more vulnerable to infection. Supplementation with immune system enhancing vitamins and minerals can help us overcome this lowered immune resistance and help us fight infections naturally.

CHAPTER 8

BACTERIAL SUPPLEMENTATION

Healthy Flora, A Healthy Body

Bacterial supplements are extremely beneficial to your health. The most important action of bacterial supplements is their reinforcement of the population of the billions of "good" bacteria that live within the body. In medical terms, these billions of bacteria are referred to as the body's bacterial flora. This chapter begins by illustrating the importance of maintaining a healthy bacterial flora and goes on to discuss how bacterial supplements can help you to do so safely and easily. It also discusses how bacterial supplements work in your body and, finally, it provides guidelines for their use.

THE IMPORTANCE OF HEALTHY BACTERIAL FLORA

The skin, the digestive tract, and the vagina in females are colonized by billions of bacteria that are essential for the proper functioning of these organs. The greatest number of bacteria are found in the digestive tract, where up to 500 species reside. Collectively, these bacteria are referred to as the intestinal flora. They are responsible for numerous important activities, some of which are closely linked to immune function, nutritional status, and detoxification of the body.

The quality of our intestinal flora is determined by the balance between the various species of bacteria within our bodies. Each species keeps the others in check, preventing the overgrowth of any one species by producing certain organic acids, which makes the environment inhospitable to harmful bacteria. This ecological balance can be disturbed by factors such as diet, chronic stress, surgery, major temperature changes, and drugs such as antibiotics.

Maintaining healthy bacterial flora in the intestine has a number of beneficial effects. Let's look more closely at some of these.

Intestinal Flora and Colon Cancer

Many studies have shown that the incidence of colon cancer is very low among vegetarians but high among meat eaters. Stool samples from strict vegetarians have a significantly higher population of lactobacilli bacteria *(Lactobacillus acidophilus)*—the good guys! Eating meat favors an increase in putrefactive bacteria, such as the bacteriodes—the bad guys—and a decrease in lactobacilli. These putrefactive bacteria have the potential to produce chemicals, such as toxic amines, that can damage the lining of the colon, ultimately forming a cancerous growth. Since lactobacilli protect against this, it is important to take them on a daily basis as a preventative measure against colon cancer. It has also been demonstrated that good bacteria are important during the treatment of colon cancer. Neumeister (1969) showed that supplements of the two bacteria found in live yogurt—*Lactobacillus acidophilus* and *Bifidobacterium bifidus,* often shortened to acidophilus and bifidus, respectively—taken during irradiation therapy reduced the side-effects of this therapy by 40 percent. Other studies have confirmed this, so I recommend the use of a beneficial bacterial culture, such as live yogurt, during radiation therapy and chemotherapy for the treatment of cancer.

Intestinal Flora and Calcium Absorption

The absorption of calcium through the wall of the intestine into the bloodstream is enhanced by healthy intestinal flora. Calcium absorption is enhanced in an acidic environment, such as the type produced by beneficial bacteria. This is particularly important when osteoporosis may be a concern, especially in postmenopausal women who do not exercise much and who have a low calcium content in their diet. Taking live yogurt daily can aid calcium absorption and help prevent osteoporosis.

Intestinal Flora and Cholesterol

Several studies have shown that the consumption of good bacteria, such as acidophilus, causes a reduction in serum cholesterol levels (Mann and Spoerry, 1974; Mann, 1977). In addition, infants who were fed a milk formula supplemented with lactobacilli were shown to have lower levels of blood cholesterol than those to whom milk without lactobacilli was fed. Laboratory studies performed on piglets that were fed a high cholesterol diet yielded similar results. These studies verify that taking good bacteria, like those found in live yogurt, can reduce the level of blood cholesterol and, therefore, reduce the risk of heart disease.

Intestinal Flora and Constipation and Diarrhea

In a healthy person, "good" bacteria—for example those found in live yogurt (acidophilus and bifidus)—produce acids, such as lactic acid, that keep the environment around them acidic. Both constipation and diarrhea can be treated with live yogurt. Numerous medical researchers have shown the beneficial effects lactobacilli—either as live yogurt or in the form of freeze-dried capsules—have on bowel movements.

Good bacteria play a very important role in digestion. For example, the higher the percentage of these good bacteria in the digestive tract, the more peristalsis—natural contractions of the digestive tract—is stimulated. Peristalsis flushes out waste material in the stool. Regular bowel movements are important for everyone, but are even more essential in old age. The consumption of live yogurt by the elderly population has benefits not only for the bowel but also for the body in general. Also, the calcium in yogurt is a protection against osteoporosis.

Diarrhea is a frequent problem for travelers. They often suffer from all kinds of gastrointestinal problems, particularly infections like gastroenteritis, which can turn into a long-lasting infection. Taking lactobacilli prior to and during a vacation can protect you from diseases caused by intestinal pathogens.

Intestinal Flora and Antibiotic Therapy

Therapy with any antibiotic, particularly broad-spectrum antibiotics, such as amoxicillin, tetracycline, and ampicillin, and the long-term use of antibiotics, as in the treatment of acne, are liable to alter the balance of the intestinal flora. Very strong antibiotics, such as clindamycin may cause drastic changes. If, for example, the body's bacterial flora are partly destroyed by taking an antibiotic, harmful bacteria can replace the good bacteria that have been destroyed.

Taking antibiotics orally often causes gastrointestinal disturbances, especially in young children. Many complain of vague symptoms such as nausea, a dull ache, and a sickly feeling all over the abdomen. Diarrhea is probably the most common side effect of antibiotic therapy; however, it can also result in flatulence, bloating, and loss of appetite. Long-term problems can range from allergies, recurrent infections, and irritable bowel syndrome to more serious problems such as diabetes, liver damage, and chronic candidiasis, also known as intestinal thrush.

Certain antibiotics, like amoxicillin, can upset the bacterial flora of the bowel and vagina. In both of these regions, a yeast infection called thrush, which is caused by *Candida albicans*, can develop. A thrush infection is most apparent in the vagina, as it produces a visible discharge; it is less apparent in the bowel, as few or no symptoms are present initially.

In a healthy person, "good" bacteria, such as those found in live yogurt, (acidophilus and bifidus) produce acids, such as lactic acid. Harmful bacteria and yeast, such as those responsible for thrush, cannot grow in an acidic environment. They can, however, grow in an environment whose acidity has been decreased. This can happen when certain drugs are taken—antibiotics and the contraceptive pill in particular. These drugs alter the natural bacterial flora lining the digestive and genital tracts, which can result in a chronic infection of these organs with harmful bacteria, yeast, or fungi.

Because of the increased susceptibility to illness after antibiotic therapy, it is very important to re-establish the normal intestinal flora as soon as possible. In the 1950s, doctors used to advise their patients to use a bacterial culture while taking a course of antibiotics. Today, that practice has stopped, even though many more antibiotics are being taken and stronger ones are being used much more commonly.

When on a course of antibiotics, take a supplement of "good" bacteria, preferably acidophilus in combination with bifidus. This will protect you against many gastro-intestinal side effects.

Intestinal Flora and Essential Vitamins

Live cultures of lactobacilli, as in fermented milk products like live yogurt, have high levels of folic acid and most B vitamins. What remains in doubt is how much of these vitamins are actually absorbed across the wall of the intestine and therefore used in the body.

Lactobacilli in the intestine manufacture vitamin K_2. This vitamin is required for the formation of substances necessary for the clotting of blood in the liver. Hence, the body is dependent on bacteria in the intestine to manufacture enough vitamin K_2 to ensure normal blood clotting. A vitamin K deficiency can result in nose bleeds, excessive bruising, blood in the urine (haematuria), and excessive menstrual blood loss. Fortunately, some vitamin K is present in green vegetables as vitamin K_1. So even if the bacterial flora in the bowel are disturbed, if you are eating plenty of green vegetables, you may not develop a vitamin K deficiency.

It is common to see a vitamin K deficiency in newborn infants, as they have no lactobacilli in the intestine to synthesize this vitamin. Most hospitals give babies one milligram of vitamin K at birth as a prophylactic measure against the development of spontaneous bleeding—further testimony to the importance of a healthy bacterial population in the digestive tract.

Intestinal Flora and Bowel Infections

There is now conclusive scientific evidence to show that lactobacilli produce substances that inhibit the growth of microbial pathogens—disease-causing organisms. The use of lactobacilli as dietary supplements has been found to alleviate intestinal infections in humans as well as animals (Shahani and Ayebo, 1980). Lactobacilli produce certain organic acids called biocines, which can kill off invading pathogens or inhibit their growth. *Lactobacillus acidophilus* is one species of lactobacilli, and it produces several biocines, such as acidophilin, lactocidin, and acidolin (Hamdan et al., 1973).

Intestinal Flora and the Immune System

The digestive tract serves as an interface beween the internal environment of the body and the external world, as it opens to the external world to take in food and to eliminate wastes. For this reason, it must be lined with billions of bacteria, which act as a first line of defense. These beneficial bacteria help fight against foreign microbes that may be ingested, thereby making them part of the immune system. If this flora is damaged, one will be made more susceptible to infection by invading bacteria, fungi, viruses, and parasites.

WAYS TO SUPPLEMENT WITH BACTERIA

You now know just how important the proper balance of bacterial flora is to your health. You have also seen how this balance can be thrown off kilter. Fortunately, the use of bacterial supplements can ensure that your body maintains strong, well-balanced, bacterial colonies. Let's look at three types of supplements that can easily be added to your diet or your supplement regimen.

Live Yogurt

If you knew how important it is to consume live yogurt, you would be eating barrels of it every day! If you want to avoid all kinds of health problems, from constipation to bowel cancer, eat a container or two—approximately twelve ounces— of live yogurt daily! The reason it is so important and useful to your health is that it contains the bacterial cultures *Lactobacillus bulgaricus* and *Streptococcus thermophilus*. These are found in most fermented milk products, including buttermilk. Live yogurt also contains *Lactobacillus acidophilus* and *Bifidobacterium bifidus*.

Yogurts containing live bacterial cultures are not heat-treated after the bacterial cultures are added. Therefore, the live bacterial cultures are able to survive in the intestine and multiply. Most commercial yogurts are heat-treated, which kills the beneficial live cultures. So the majority of commercial yogurts do not have the same therapeutic value as yogurts that contain a living culture. Use only yogurt that clearly indicates that it has a live culture of any of the above-mentioned bacteria. Yogurt with live cultures will clot or curd within twenty-four hours.

Whey

Whey is a byproduct of the manufacture of cheese, and contains live bacterial cultures similar to those in live yogurt. When the fat and protein are removed from milk to make cheese, whey remains. It contains a high concentration of lactic acid and milk enzymes. Acids, such as lactic acid, maintain a low pH level (acidic environment) in the bowel and kill off any overgrowth of unhealthy bacteria and fungi; the low pH also stimulates peristalsis, allowing for regular bowel motions.

As it is acidic, whey is a natural antiseptic. It is an excellent remedy for sore throats and inflammation of the mucous membranes of the nose and throat. "Whey cures" were famous throughout Europe in the nineteenth century, and many, including royalty, used to visit the health spas of Switzerland to undergo a whey cure. Whey cures were used to treat a whole range of disorders, including constipation, pancreatic problems, hormonal problems, obesity, and circulatory problems, such as blocked arteries.

Like live yogurt, whey should be taken on a regular basis; especially if there are bowel problems such as flatulence, constipation, alteration in the bowel habit, alteration in the bacterial population, diverticulitis, colitis, and chronic bowel infections. Over the last six years, I have treated these intestinal disorders and can support what Swiss doctors have been saying for many years about the importance of whey and yogurt.

If taking whey internally, put a teaspoonful to a tablespoonful in an eight-ounce glass of water and take with each meal. This will regulate the secretion of acid from the stomach, as well as assist the colon in efficient functioning. Since whey is a byproduct of cheese-making, it can be obtained from farms where cheese is manufactured. It can also be obtained commercially in some health-food shops. Molkosan, made by Bioforce, is a product produced by Dr. Alfred Vogel, the famous Swiss naturopath, and it is an excellent source of whey. Another popular whey supplement is Whey to Go from Solgar.

Bacterial Supplements in Capsule Form

For the most part, live yogurt is made from cow's milk, although it can also be made from sheep's or goat's milk. Anyone who does not want to take fermented milk in the form of live yogurt can take a bacterial supplement in the form of freeze-dried capsules instead. These capsules contain the beneficial bacteria *Lactobacillus acidophilus,* either by itself or in combination with other bacteria such as *Bifidobacterium bifidus.* These tablets are sold in most health food shops and pharmacies under the names Acidophilus, Biodophilus, and Multidophilus.

While these tablets are excellent, I always prefer to recommend what nature provides—fermented milk. However, I am aware that some people, particularly children, find it difficult to take live yogurt, while still others are allergic to cow's milk. For these people, the freeze-dried capsules are an excellent alternative. If using capsules, keep them in a cool place and remember that once opened, capsules last for only about three weeks. They should be replaced after this time.

USING A BACTERIAL SUPPLEMENT EFFECTIVELY

There are a few diet-related factors to consider when using a bacterial supplement. Bacteria are sensitive to temperature, so try not to take either very cold or very hot food or drinks together with the supplement. It is best not to take a bacterial supplement (except whey) with food at all. Take your supplement on an empty stomach—at least one hour before a meal or two hours after. However, if you must take your supplement just before or after a meal, be sure that meal does not contain protein, as protein may slow the food's transit time, allowing it to remain in the acidic stomach too long. This

Nutritional Medicine at Work

A number of my patients with bowel problems have experienced great relief from using bacterial supplements. Jane is a good example of one of these patients. She came to me complaining of diarrhea alternating with periods of constipation, bloating, and abdominal cramps, especially after eating. She told me that her husband would complain that her tummy was "rumbling and grumbling" all night long. She herself was very aware of the gurgling noises in her intestine, and it was a source of great embarrassment to her.

Jane had been on the contraceptive pill continuously for five years. She had also taken tetracycline and doxycycline during the past year, each for three months, as treatment for acne.

I suspected a disturbance of the intestinal flora for three reasons: her symptoms; her use of two broad-spectrum antibiotics—both of which are known to cause gross disturbance of the intestinal flora; and her use of the contraceptive pill, which is also known to upset intestinal flora. Laboratory tests revealed a low percentage of lactobacilli in the stool. Her dietary history also revealed that she had a high intake of processed foods and a very low intake of fresh vegetables and fruit.

I asked Jane to increase her intake of fresh fruit and vegetables and recommended a bacterial supplement—live yogurt, in this case. She was to take this daily over a three-month period in addition to one tablespoon of whey in a glass of water with each meal. With these simple measures, her bowel habits returned to normal and the bloating and cramps disappeared. In Jane's case, no medicine was necessary. This surprised even me, as I suspected from her initial visit that I would have to use tetracycline injeel, a homeopathic medicine used to undo the harmful effects of tetracycline in the body. Jane proved the point that simple measures often work best if given time, and that good food is often the best medicine of all.

increases the exposure of the bacterial supplements to stomach acid, which can kill the bacteria. The faster the bacterial supplement gets out of the stomach and into the small intestine, the greater the number of bacteria that will survive to benefit your health.

Bacterial supplements are important to your health. The benefits of having a high concentration of helpful bacteria in the bowel are numerous and include improved digestion, improved immunity, and reduced risk of bowel disease, such as cancer.

Of all bacterial supplements, live yogurt is perhaps the most important. But when it is not possible or wise to use live yogurt, other bacterial supplements can give you the benefits of this food, allowing you to maintain good health in one of the easiest and safest ways.

CHAPTER 9

HEALTHY DIET—A FORM OF NUTRITIONAL MEDICINE

Healthy Food Is the Best Medicine

Eating and breathing are the two most important things we do every day in order to stay alive. The food you nourish your body with is of critical importance to your health. The right diet can keep you healthy, preventing infection and limiting the amount of medication you'll need to take in your lifetime. Good food—natural foods that nature intended you to eat—will provide your body with the nutrients essential for good health, particularly an effective immune system. Bad food—unnatural or processed foods—will not.

After spending twelve years in Africa, I returned to Europe and was shocked to see the kind of food that people in Europe and the United States were eating. In Africa, people eat a diet based on natural foods, at least for the most part. The diet generally consists of high roughage foods, such as yams, maize meal, vegetables, and occasional meat. This simpler diet ensures that there are less toxic additives and encourages better bowel habits, both of which enhance one's level of health. In Europe and the United States, much of the food that is consumed is "dead" food. It contains too much sugar and much of it is processed. This introduction of foreign chemicals increases the level of toxins in the body. The lack of roughage in the diet also slows waste elimination from the body, allowing the toxins to remain in the body longer.

This chapter will explain why natural food is beneficial to our health, present guidelines for a healthy diet, and consider some foods that can actually compromise your health.

THE BENEFITS OF A NATURAL DIET

All energy on this planet comes from the sun. The sun provides us with heat and light energy. As Figure 9.1 shows, plants use light energy from the sun to make food in a beautiful process called photosynthesis. During photosynthesis, light energy is converted to chemical energy. This energy is passed along to us when we eat the plant. In an indirect way then, energy from the sun ends up in our bodies when we eat plants, helping to keep us healthy. Hence, we refer to natural foods as being energy-rich. Humans are part of an energy pathway. It is no small wonder then that so many cultures have worshipped the sun, as it is truly the giver of life on this planet.

Much of the food we eat, however, is removed from the energy pathway shown above, and processed in a factory. Unnatural chemicals are often added, such as flavorings, colorings, or preservatives. The food is depleted of its natural energy; it is "dead," so to speak. It is also toxic for the body,

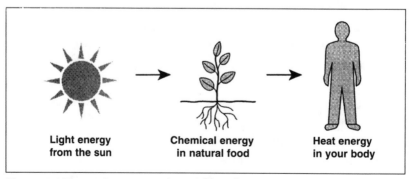

Figure 9.1 Energy being transferred from the sun to you.

due to the presence of these additives. The liver then has to detoxify these chemicals and send them to the kidneys, which excretes them. This puts a greater workload on these organs. The message is simple—the closer your food is to nature, the higher its energy content and the healthier your body will be for eating it.

GUIDELINES FOR A HEALTHY DIET

As stated earlier, eating is one of the most important things that we do to stay alive. What we choose to eat has a great effect on our health. One of our primary concerns, then, should be taking notice of what we eat. Unfortunately, all too often, we neglect this concern. Following, you will find some important guidelines for healthy eating that will help you to keep your body—your immune system in particular—healthy.

The Importance of a Low-Fat, High-Fiber Diet

Today, most people know the importance of reducing their fat intake. Not only is it necessary for reducing your waist-line, it is also necessary for your health. A high-fat diet has been implicated as a causative factor in cancer, cardiovascular diseases, and diabetes. What many do not know, however, is the importance of combining a low-fat diet with a high-fiber intake.

A low-fat, high-fiber diet has been proven to reduce one's risk of degenerative diseases, as well as to improve one's overall health. Soluble fiber helps move food through your digestive system quickly, preventing it from remaining in the system for too long, thereby improving your overall health.

One can obtain fiber through fresh fruits and vegetables and whole grains. It is recommended that one consume at least 25 grams of dietary fiber per day. Most Americans, however, fall far short of this goal due to the refining process of grains that is so common in this country. While whole brown rice and whole wheat are excellent sources of fiber, white rice and refined white flour are stripped of their fiber, as well as essential vitamins and minerals. Even fortified rice and flour are devoid of fiber and many nutrients that they once had before they were stripped.

Fruits and Vegetables—The Importance of Five to Seven a Day

While it is recommended that individuals eat *at least* five to seven servings of fruits and vegetables per day, most Americans consume no more than three to five servings. This is highly unfortunate, since fruits and vegetables offer untold amounts of vitamins, minerals, fiber, and phytochemicals— compounds that have disease-protective effects in the body. Your overall healthy diet should include a *minimum* of five to seven servings of vegetables per day.

The Importance of Water

Water is the body's single most important nutrient. Approximately 60 percent of the human body consists of water. Almost all of the body's functions rely on water—water maintains the body's temperature at 98.6°F, carries nutrients to the cells, carries waste and toxins away from the cells and out of the body, and provides protection and cushioning for the joints and organs of the body. In the course of a day, water is lost through breathing, sweating, and elimination. The body does not maintain an extra store of water as it does other nutrients, however, so it is important that we replenish the body's supply of water by taking in fluids. It is generally recommended that a healthy adult drink one and a half to two quarts of water per day. This is just a guideline. The most important thing is to listen to your own body. When you are thirsty, drink water—but make sure it's safe water! Filtered or fresh spring water is best, although bottled water is better than tap water. This is because, unfortunately, water—the most basic of all nutrients—is now becoming unsafe to drink.

The quality of our water supplies has become a major public health issue. In many cities, tap water is not only foul-tasting and foul-smelling, it also contains additives, such as chlorine, fluoride, heavy metals, and various other chemicals that can be potentially harmful to the body. Chlorine is used to kill harmful bacteria in the water supply, but it also kills some of the "good" bacteria in the human digestive system and has been found to provoke asthma attacks and contribute to arteriosclerosis (hardening of the arteries). Fluoride, another substance commonly added to the water supply, has been shown to be detrimental to the body. According to Bernard Jensen and Mark Andersen in *Empty Harvest*, sodium fluoride adversely affects our enzymes and thyroid glands, leading to problems with immunity and other health problems. It creates a high incidence of bone fractures as well.

In 1974, a Safe Drinking Water Act was passed in the United States. Since that time, many contaminants have been found in water; 97 percent of these contaminants are believed to cause cancer, 82 percent are believed to cause birth defects, and 23 percent are believed to promote the growth of tumors. For these reasons, the importance of using either filtered or bottled water cannot be stressed enough.

FOODS TO BE AVOIDED

Just as there are foods that are beneficial to our health, there are those that are detrimental. Following is a discussion of foods that, in addition to not being of benefit to your health, should actually be avoided.

Sugar

Refined sugar, like refined flour, is a product of Western civilization. It's an unnatural food and so, completely unnecessary in the diet. Your body is a natural organism that requires natural foods to function efficiently. Eating unnatural foods goes against nature. Worse still, it contributes to ill health.

Sugar contains absolutely no nutrients, so even small amounts are not at all *necessary* in the diet; in fact, consumption of too much sugar can actually deplete your body of several vitamins and minerals.

Over 150 years ago, Native American Indians warned of the harmful effects of refined sugar on the body. They observed that Westernized cultures ate too many sweet things, which weakened the body. Today their words are proving to be all too true. Among the adults that I see, there is almost an epidemic of fungal infections, skin rashes, and intestinal candidiasis. Many of these infections improve when sugar and foods that contain sugar are excluded from the diet.

Sugar encourages the growth of a number of bacteria and fungi—it is a wonderful growth medium for these microorganisms. As a result, a diet rich in sweet things may predispose a person to infections. Sugar consumption is associated with tooth decay, candidiasis, and mucus production, especially in people predisposed to respiratory problems, such as asthmatics. Sugar can also increase your threshold for sweetness, causing you to lose your taste for more natural foods. Many people are now addicted to sugar. As with cigarettes, it can become very difficult to live without it.

In one study by Sanchez et al. (1973), a high intake of sugar was found to have a negative effect on the immune system. This study showed that sugar impaired the ability of white blood cells to gobble up and kill bacteria. This research followed the work of an American physician named Dr. Sandler who, while working with victims of the polio epidemic in the late 1940s, became convinced that a high sugar intake made one more susceptible to this disease. The 1973 research supported Dr. Sandler's hypothesis, as refined sugar was clearly found to suppress the immune system. Other studies have shown that sugar robs the body of certain nutrients, including zinc, which is vital for immune function.

The amount of sugar consumed by the average adult and

child in the Western world is indeed troubling. When shopping in American supermarkets, it is alarming to see just how many of the foods on the shelves contain sugar. Most breakfast cereals contain sugar—even a bowl of cereal that is considered "healthy," such as muesli, may contain the equivalent of two tablespoons of sugar. Soft drinks also have a high sugar content—Coca-Cola contains the equivalent of seven teaspoons of sugar per six-ounce glass! These examples show how important it is to read the labels on all processed foods. If you wish to know the quantity of any of the specific constituents of a particular food item, write to the manufacturer.

Sugar has a detrimental effect on everyone's health, but it especially affects the health of children, who often consume excessive amounts it. Many of the children attending my clinic suffer from recurrent infections, asthma, and eczema. An alarming number of them are also deficient in various minerals. The first thing I recommend for these children is a reduction in sugar intake. Some are in such a poor state of health that it is necessary to cut out all sugars for a limited period, thereby allowing their young bodies to recover from the ill effects of too much sugar. The benefits of this treatment are almost immediate. There is an increase in both appetite and energy levels. The whole body begins to function better.

The body is disturbed by the ups and downs that occur in the blood sugar level when sugary foods are consumed. These ups and downs put stress on the pancreas and the adrenal glands, causing the latter to secrete adrenaline, which causes the blood sugar level to drop below normal, a condition known as hypoglycemia. When eaten only occasionally, sugary foods do not cause too much difficulty—it is only when the pancreas and adrenal glands are constantly stressed that problems arise. Avoid such difficulties by only eating natural foods and by avoiding sugars that have been bleached or chemically refined and therefore rendered harmful to the body.

Look at the two graphs in Figure 9.2. When natural foods

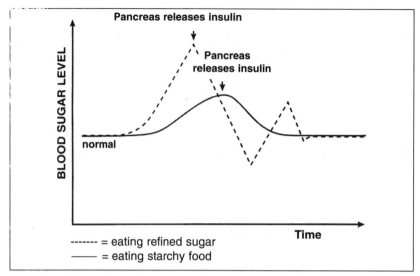

Figure 9.2 The effects of sugar on blood sugar levels

containing starch, such as potatoes and rice, are eaten, the
blood sugar (glucose) level rises gradually, as the solid line
indicates. When the blood sugar level reaches a certain point,
the pancreas releases insulin, which regulates glucose levels,
and the blood sugar level slowly drops back to normal. In
contrast to this, eating sweets or any foods rich in refined
sugar causes high levels of glucose to enter the bloodstream
rapidly, as the dashed line indicates. This puts stress on the
pancreas, forcing it to release large quantities of insulin, as
too much sugar in the bloodstream can be dangerous (hyper-
glycemia).

At public talks, I am often asked, "Doesn't the body need
sugar?" The answer is: "Yes, it does." The body does, in fact,
require certain types of natural sugar in order to function.
The process through which the body processes sugar provides the body with energy and heat. Glucose—the form of
sugar found in the blood—is required for the cells of the body
to function properly. The body does not, however, benefit
from unnatural sugars, such as dextrose and sucrose, taken in
large quantities on a regular basis. While the body needs a

certain amount of natural sugar, such as fructose, in order to function, it is able to produce sugar for itself by converting carbohydrates—found in grains, starches, and certain vegetables—into glucose. Refined sugar, however, is in no way necessary to your diet.

If a sweetener is desired, the best sugar is always the sugar that can be found in natural foods—especially in fresh or dried fruits. Raisins and dates are all very sweet and can be used instead of sugar to sweeten breakfast cereal. Also, the sugar in fruit and honey—fructose—is natural and much healthier than refined sugar.

Sodium

While small amounts of sodium are necessary for the body, sodium is one mineral whose intake needs to be limited rather than increased. Too much sodium, combined with a low intake of potassium, can lead to high blood pressure and weakened bones. The average American diet probably contains more sodium than is necessary. Sodium intake should be limited to 2,400 milligrams per day. However, most prepared foods contain large amounts of sodium, and this requirement can be fulfilled in one meal. If you avoid prepackaged foods and using table salt in your cooking and as a seasoning, you can limit your intake to 2,400 mg a day. There are also low-sodium alternatives in packaged foods now available.

Processed Foods

Nature did not intend us to eat from bottles, tins, jars, or packets. The body likes food it can digest and absorb into the bloodstream easily. It likes to receive not only protein, carbohydrate, and fat in this form, but also vitamins and minerals in forms that are easily absorbed. Putting natural foods into a natural system like the human body makes sense. Ingesting unnatural chemicals, such as those found in processed foods, does not make sense.

During the 1950s and 1960s, processed foods became part of that dubious package called "progress" that was sold to people in the West. The country market was replaced by the supermarket in the belief that bigger was better. Even the supermarkets grew up to become mega-supermarkets. Remember that the primary aim of the food processing industry is profit, not health! It is encouraging to see that country markets are springing up again and that the availability of organically grown foods is increasing. This trend must be encouraged for the sake of ourselves and our children. Put pressure on your local supermarket and grocer to supply organically grown foods.

The best quality cereals, fruits, and vegetables come from organic farms—farms that allow the soil time to replenish itself between crop cycles and do not use chemical fertilizers, chemical pesticides, or chemical herbicides.

You can now begin to see why it is important to know how and where your fruits and vegetables are grown. If in doubt, either grow your own produce or buy produce that has been organically grown.

In addition to the importance of eating the right foods, it is also important to eat correctly. Never eat when stressed or while doing something else. Set time aside that is reserved only for eating meals. Also be sure to chew your food slowly and well. Fasting for three days once a month is also a good practice for cleansing the system.

I knew very little about nutrition upon leaving medical school. Most of what I've learned since then has been from courses I have taken on natural medicine, mainly in Austria. I once thought of nutrition as unimportant and less exciting than pharmacology—the use of drugs. Today, however, I realize that apart from breathing, the most important thing we do every day is eat. What we put into our bodies is of the utmost importance. Nutrition should occupy a prime place in medical education.

Drinking sufficient water every day as well as cutting down on, or cutting out, sugary and processed foods will benefit your health tremendously. Remember—healthy food and water are the best medicines available!

CHAPTER 10

STRESS AND THE IMMUNE SYSTEM

The Physical Is Merely an Expression of the Spiritual

As you have seen, there are many factors that contribute to maintaining a healthy immune system. Thus far you have read about how proper diet and supplementation can keep your immune system strong. Yet another important factor is your mental and emotional state. Negative emotions have powerful effects on the physical body, primarily through the immune system. Impaired immune function can result in serious infections, autoimmune diseases, cancer, and premature death.

Stress is perhaps the most common assault to our mental state—many people find themselves under stress on a daily basis. In this chapter, you will learn about the ways stress, and the way you respond to stress, can affect your immune system. Some ideas about how to deal with the stresses in your life are also discussed.

Stress-related illness has reached epidemic proportions in the modern world. In many rural areas, however, stress is virtually nonexistent. When I was living in Africa, I found it interesting that members of the rural black community, among whom high blood pressure and heart disease are very rare, began to show signs of hypertension and heart disease as soon as they moved into towns and cities. The same pattern may be observed in any population, though. This indicates that the stresses of modern life can have damaging effects on the body.

Many people suffer from chronic stress as the result of various situations. It is important to become aware of the various stresses in your life and their effects on you. The Holmes and Rahe rating scale, found on page 147, is a popular method of measuring stress. Although it is not comprehensive—it refers to only the social aspects of your life—it is useful to relate this scale to your own life, as it will roughly assess the degree of stress you might be experiencing. Various events are rated numerically, according to their potential for causing disease. Circle those life events that you are currently enduring, and add up their mean values. A score of 200 or more is considered to be predictive of a serious illness.

EMOTIONAL RESPONSE TO STRESS

The way that you respond to stress on an emotional or mental level is important to staying healthy. In a Carnegie Mellon University study, 47 percent of those who were subjected to high levels of stress became ill. But 53 percent remained well. Both psychologists and medical scientists have been looking for reasons why some people do not get infections despite having been exposed to a virus or bacteria. The results of some studies suggest that the negative physical effects of stress can be tempered by a positive emotional response. This is further proof of the correlation between the health of mind and body.

Optimism Versus Pessimism

In 1989, Doctors D. Sobel and R. Ornstein wrote a book entitled *Healthy Pleasures*, in which they give details of their research into two groups of people—those they labeled as pessimists and those they labeled optimists. This research

Table 10.1 The Holmes and Rahe Rating Scale—
Top Twenty Events

Rank	Life Event	Mean Value
1	Death of spouse/partner	100
2	Divorce	73
3	Separation	65
4	Time spent in jail	63
5	Death of a close family member	63
6	Personal illness or injury	53
7	Marriage	50
8	Fired from job	47
9	Reconciliation with partner/spouse	45
10	Retirement	45
11	Change in family member's health	44
12	Pregnancy	40
13	Sexual problems	39
14	New member in family	39
15	Adjustments at work	39
16	Change in financial status	38
17	Death of a close friend	37
18	Changing jobs	36
19	Increased arguing with spouse/partner	35
20	Large mortgage	31

showed that optimists enjoy better immune function than do pessimists. Why? Optimists were shown to have higher numbers of so-called helper cells, a type of white blood cell that stimulates immune function, than they had of a type of cell that suppresses immune function. The higher the number of helper cells, the better one's resistance to infection will be. It is interesting to see that a person's mental state can influence their physical response to infection.

Stress and Anger

Research into the ways in which the emotional state affects an individual's response to stress ranks anger as the single most powerful suppresser of immune function, predisposing a person not only to infection but to a whole host of other illnesses, as well (Angier, 1990). Many studies now show that anger can contribute to heart disease and a range of other problems, including death.

Dr. Mara Julius of the University of Michigan looked at the effects of deep-seated anger on the health of a group of women over an eighteen-year period. Each woman was asked to complete a questionnaire specifically designed to detect suppressed anger. The most startling aspect of this study was the fact that three times as many women with a high score on the questionnaire—those with high levels of anger—died during the eighteen-year study period than those who had little or no suppressed anger.

These findings agree with those of Dr. Michael Schmidt and his coworkers as stated in the book *Beyond Antibiotics*:

Anger and hostility eat away at the substance of the human psyche. These emotions foster an atmosphere of negativity that clouds every human endeavor. Researchers are increasingly showing a link between anger, hostility, and cynicism and the development of disease and premature death.

Anyone who has participated in my workshops on stress already knows my opinions on the roles anger and fear play in human disease. In my practice, I've seen a very close link between ill health and an unhealthy emotional state. In both Ireland and South Africa, the two countries in which I have spent most of my life, I have seen overwhelming evidence that suppressed anger is the main obstacle not only to physical health, but also to growth and development as a human being.

Stress Reduction at Work

André was a young man—22 years of age—when I first met him in South Africa. He had been admitted to the hospital ten times in the course of six months with severe asthma. Twice he "died" in the emergency room and had to be resuscitated.

When André came to see me, I was alarmed by two things. First, there was the disturbing amount of medication that he was taking to control the asthma attacks. Second, there was the large number of times he had been admitted to the hospital. I suspected that this young man was in danger on a physical level, and that the cause could probably be traced to an emotional level.

André was not consciously aware of any major emotional stresses in his life when I questioned him. The real story came from his mother at a later date. Prior to being adopted, André had suffered great physical abuse from his biological parents. When they were young children, he and his brothers and sisters were locked in cupboards for days at a time. They were starved, beaten, and burned with cigarette butts. The children were eventually rescued by social workers and placed in foster care.

Because André was very young at the time of his abuse, as an adult he was unaware of much of this information; it was locked away in his subconscious. I believe, however, that it triggered a pattern of behavior when he encountered stress in a relationship, such as a fight with a girlfriend. Upon further questioning, it was revealed that all of André's severe asthma attacks were preceded by the emotional stress of an argument or disagreement with a loved one—girlfriend, mother, or father. He perceived anything that seemed to threaten these relationships as a threat to his survival. The inner turmoil he felt at such times was probably too painful to deal with, and manifested itself in the form of an asthma attack.

Using physical medicines may have been helpful to André, but it was apparent that his real need was for help at an emotional level. I am pleased to say that he is now undergoing psychotherapy with a clinical psychologist. He has not seen the inside of a hospital for the last eighteen months, and we have been able to reduce most of his conventional medicine.

André had a high level of anger that was directed against his biological parents. It was only by releasing this anger that he was able to break the cycle of hospital admissions that had brought him to me in the first place. I could quote many other similar cases, but it suffices to say that you should never underestimate the role your emotions play in determining the state of your physical health. I believe that the single biggest advancement that can be made, not just for improving one's immune system, but for one's total health, is the release of anger.

PHYSICAL RESPONSE TO STRESS

Stress can have a very negative effect on the body. Most importantly, it can impair your body's immune function, making you more susceptible to infection and disease.

During the 1920s, Professor Hans Selye of the University of Prague, carried out research into the negative effects of stress on the body. His years of research led him to propose Figure 10.1, which explains how chronic, or prolonged, stress can affect us.

Professor Selye proposed that stress can cause imbalances within the endocrine, or hormonal, system of the body—including the hypothalamus, pituitary, thyroid, thymus, and adrenal glands, the pancreas, the ovaries, and the testes—which, in turn, can suppress the immune system. This theory has been supported more recently by other medical researchers. Dr. Carl Simonton, for example, who is famous for his pioneering work with cancer patients, proposed that a high percentage of these patients had experienced a period of chronic stress preceding the onset of cancer. Simonton suggested that stress was causing a suppression of the immune system, thereby allowing cancer to develop.

How exactly does stress affect the immune system? Stress increases output from the adrenal glands, causing a rise in the levels of the hormones adrenaline and cortisone in the body. These hormones can suppress white blood cells. Since one of the most important functions of white blood cells is the destruction of invading viruses, bacteria, and fungi, it is easy to see how stress can lead to impaired immune function. In addition, a prolonged elevation of cortisone has been specifically linked to the destruction of T-lymphocytes, the so-called "killer cells" that appear to play a major role in helping the body fight cancer. The level of immune suppression is proportional to both the duration of stress and the level of stress.

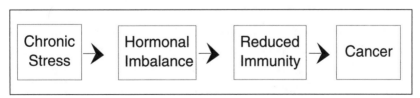

Figure 10.1 The negative effects of stress

Studies of the common cold have lent strong support to the theory that stress affects immune function. Experiments done at Oxford University in the 1970s showed that people under stress, such as business managers constantly facing deadlines, were much more susceptible to the common cold.

Other research done at Carnegie Mellon University showed that among individuals exposed to one of five common cold viruses, 47 percent of those under high levels of stress became ill, while only 27 percent of those experiencing low stress levels became sick. The doctors conducting this study suggested that " . . . stress is associated with the suppression of a general resistance process . . . leaving persons susceptible to infectious agents" (Cohen et al., 1991).

PROTECTING AGAINST THE HARMFUL EFFECTS OF STRESS

The best way to protect your immune system from the harmful effects of stress is to avoid stressful situations altogether. As this is virtually impossible in today's world, though, you must develop coping skills for dealing with stress. Fortunately, there are several things you can do to help your body better handle the everyday stresses that you may encounter.

Exercise

Regular exercise can help protect your body from the damage caused by stress in several ways. In addition to leading to an overall increase in energy, regular exercise improves heart function, reducing heart rate, improving heart muscle tone, and reducing blood pressure. Regular exercise also reduces the output of adrenaline and cortisone from the adrenal glands in response to stress. As you learned earlier, it is these substances, when produced in excess during times of stress, that are at least partly responsible for stress-induced damage of the immune system. Through regular exercise, the oxygen uptake of all cells in the body is improved. The cells of the central nervous system consume approximately 25 percent of this oxygen uptake, so making them better able to function and cope with the negative effects of stress. Finally, exercising regularly improves your self-esteem and fosters a feeling of well-being, leaving you less susceptible to negative feelings, and, therefore, less susceptible to the negative effects of stress on your immune system.

Relaxation

Deep relaxation has been shown to have a positive effect on immune function. One particular scientific reference has shown that powerful immune-enhancing chemicals are released in the body during periods of deep sleep (Moldofsky et al., 1986). This supports what our common sense tells us— that deep relaxation and good-quality sleep can have a beneficial effect on our physical health, so making it easier to cope in times of stress.

Just as important, certain physiological changes occur in the body that make it easier to handle stress. To begin, heart rate is reduced and blood pressure is lowered, both of which help you to remain calm in the face of stress. There is also better movement of blood from the peripheries of the body towards the internal organs. When you are relaxed, your sweat production is reduced, and your digestion is improved, due to increased secretion of digestive juices. Finally, during deep relaxation, you have a shallow, calmer breathing rate. All of these physiological responses help your body to better cope in the face of stress.

Only you know which relaxation technique is the most effective for you. You might choose a learned relaxation technique, such as meditation, progressive relaxation, self-hypnosis, visualization, or yoga. Or you might prefer a relaxing activity, such as fishing, reading, or dancing. Do what feels right for you.

Nutritional Supplementation

Because chronic stress causes a continual increase in adrenaline and cortisone secretion from the adrenal glands, these glands can become exhausted and can shrink, or atrophy. Certain nutritional supplements, such as potassium, vitamin C, vitamin B_6, pantothenic acid, zinc, and magnesium can help prevent adrenal gland damage. Hence, a good vitamin and mineral supplement is important. But be sure that the supplement contains the above ingredients. Potassium and pantothenic acid are particularly important for adrenal gland support. Foods rich in potassium include avocados, potatoes, raw tomatoes, bananas, melons, and fish. Foods that are good sources of pantothenic acid include whole grains, legumes, cauliflower, broccoli, raw tomatoes, and liver.

Korean Ginseng

The herb ginseng has been shown to protect the body against many of the harmful effects of stress, including physical and mental fatigue. In addition, it is the best herb to take to support adrenal function. Korean ginseng is an adaptogen, a substance that protects against mental and physical fatigue, provides protection against stress, and maintains a normal metabolic state in the body during the challenges of stress. It is able to function as an adaptogen partly through its action on the central nervous system and partly through its action on the adrenal glands. Ginseng appears to influence a number of the control mechanisms within the central nervous system in an effort to keep the metabolism regulated during periods of stress. Many of the historical uses of ginseng relate to its ability to nourish the adrenal glands and to protect the body in times of stress.

Ginseng can be taken as an herbal tincture, in dry form, or in homeopathic form. I prefer to use the dried root in powdered form, which I then combine with licorice to assist its absorption into the bloodstream. Put four teaspoons of powdered ginseng root and four teaspoons of licorice in a cup of water. Bring to a boil and simmer for ten minutes. Drink this two or three times a day.

Viewing Stress in a Positive Light

While it is true that stress can be detrimental to your health, stressful events can have a positive effect. In order to see this, we must focus our thoughts and energy on the positive. Stress, adversity, and change are great motivators. They teach us a great deal about ourselves. It is often easy to be overwhelmed by the negative aspects of stress. But stress precipitates a need to seek help, be it from a doctor, a psychologist, a counselor, or a friend. This sets off a sequence of events that usually results in inner growth, often in the form of a greater awareness about ourselves and everything going on around us. The story of André in the inset "Stress Reduction at Work" on page 149 is a good example of this. He was under such physical stress with his asthma that he began to seek a different way of dealing with his illness. This resulted in his seeking emotional help, and as a result, he now has a much greater understanding of his disease and how to control it— i.e., he has a much higher level of self-awareness.

Stress Management Techniques

Learning about stress management can help you to learn to better handle the stresses in your life and, as a result, help you to maintain your health. There are a variety of different stress management techniques you can try. The best stress management techniques are the ones that work for you.

Stress management addresses the deeper issues—the emotional issues behind the stress—and helps you to see the positive side of yourself, making you stronger emotionally spiritually. This can be taught in an experiential way, through doing exercises that enhance awareness.

At the stress management courses I run in conjunction with other therapists, we aim to develop a much higher level

A Positive View of Stress at Work

Three years ago, Angela, diagnosed with breast cancer which had spread to the liver and bone, came to see me. On her third visit to my office, she said that she was glad she had developed cancer! I had never heard a cancer patient say this kind of thing before, so I asked her what she meant.

She replied, "Cancer has helped me to see the beauty all around me. I have always loved flowers, but I was always too busy to spend time in my garden. I always walked through the front garden on my way to and from work, but I never found time to simply enjoy it. Because I know that I may die at any time, I now walk into the garden, touch the daffodils, smell them, talk to them—I've become aware of their beauty. Slowly, I've become aware of the beauty in trees and animals. I've become aware of the beauty inside people and wish that they could see it themselves. I've also become aware of the beauty within myself."

This was a remarkable statement from a woman who had a death sentence hanging over her. Although she had initially interpreted the diagnosis of breast cancer as frightening and negative, she was able to ease the stress of her situation by locating a positive aspect to her predicament. A diagnosis of a potentially fatal disease, such as cancer, is an understandably large source of stress for the patient. Angela, however, chose to find a positive side to her situation, and in doing so, she had developed a deep spiritual awareness of the beauty within all of us.

of self-awareness in the participants. We try to help people to become more aware through the experience of novel forms of meditation, music and dance, self-hypnosis, and visualization. We usually run these courses over weekends. This helps people to stop temporarily and remove themselves from their daily routines. We encourage them to focus on the positive side of even the most tragic events in life, and to identify and release the greatest obstacles to human happiness—anger and fear. So much human pain and sickness has its origins in one or both of these feelings. Having the courage to face these feelings and to deal with them allows enormous personal growth to take place. Participants then begin to accept themselves and to become much more comfortable and at ease, and this serves to alleviate stress.

Stress can affect the immune system, allowing recurrent infections to develop. Some of the most effective ways of counteracting stress are deep relaxation, meditation, and good quality sleep. You must also remember that a good diet and adequate supplementation are necessary. Should stress prove unavoidable, you can protect your body against the adverse effects of stress through regular exercise, adequate periods of relaxation, and the use of natural substances to support proper functioning of the adrenal glands. These should include a good mineral and vitamin supplement and Korean ginseng. The healthful effects of a positive attitude, and the ability to locate positive aspects in even the most negative of situations, cannot be overlooked either.

Someone once asked me to explain in one sentence how to overcome the stresses of modern life. My answer was, "Be yourself and stop trying to fit someone else's picture of you." When you are being yourself completely, your anxiety level drops and, as a consequence, life becomes infinitely less stressful, and much more rewarding.

CONCLUSION

The purpose of this book is to show that there are valid and effective ways to prevent and treat infections without using antibiotics. Antibiotics have only been produced commercially in the last fifty years. Prior to that, infections were treated in other ways. The knowledge that natural alternatives to antibiotics exist is becoming increasingly important as the overuse and misuse of antibiotic drugs continues to contribute to the problem of bacterial resistance to antibiotics.

Some of the methods that I use in my practice with great success have been mentioned in this book. Hopefully, they will gain more popularity in years to come. The main difficulty I've encountered is the general lack of availability of these preparations in pharmacies and health food shops. In Germany and France, it is very easy to gain access to "alternative" medicines—homeopathic, herbal, nutritional supplements, and mixtures of these—through most pharmacies. Unfortunately, this is not always the case in the United States. It is only with your support that this situation will change. Ask your local health-food store to stock some of these medicines.

I believe in the old ways of doing things, ways that are simple and natural, ways that are accessible to everyone. Today, medicines are becoming more and more expensive. Even many natural methods of healing have now become commercially oriented. Wisdom and a respect for nature do not sit comfortably beside profit-driven commercial enterprises. Yet the wisdom handed down from generation to generation is vital for our survival. This wisdom, as well as a deep respect for nature, are evident among the African tribes with whom I have lived. They are also apparent among Native American Indians.

It is encouraging to see an increasing interest in these people and their ways—especially from Westerners. I am pleased to observe and be part of this change, and to see the emergence of a more holistic view, not just of medicine, but of the entire world.

The best natural alternative to antibiotics is to maintain your health so that antibiotics are not needed. It is easy to do this naturally. You need only remember to eat a healthy diet that is low in refined sugars and processed foods; take vitamin and mineral supplements to boost your immunity and bolster your health; exercise regularly; allow your body the rest it needs; avoid stressful situations whenever possible; and, when stress cannot be avoided, try to approach it in a positive way. By doing these things, you help to ensure that your immune system is strong and healthy and, therefore, able to protect you from disease and infection.

There are times when an antibiotic is necessary to treat an infection. Before you begin taking antibiotics, though, be sure that the infection that you are treating is of a bacterial nature; antibiotics are not effective against viral infections. I also recommend that when taking an antibiotic, you also take a bacterial supplement, vitamin C, and echinacea. In doing so, you not only shorten the duration of the infection, but also protect your body against some of the side effects associated with the use of antibiotic.

I hope you have gained something from reading this book. Please write and let me know what your opinions are. Your comments will help me with future editions. I wish you and your loved ones well. May you live happy, healthy lives.

Dr. John McKenna
c/o Avery Publishing Group, Inc.
120 Old Broadway
Garden City Park, NY 11040

BIBLIOGRAPHY

Chapter 1. The History of Antibiotics

Chain, E., et al. "Penicillin as a Chemotherapeutic Agent." *The Lancet* 1 (1940): 226–228.

Conacher, Duff, and Associates. "Troubled Waters on Tap: Organic Chemicals in Public Drinking Water Systems and the Failure of Regulation." Washington, DC: Center for the Study of Responsive Law, January 1988.

Cowen, D. L. and A. B. Segelman. *Antibiotics in Historical Perspective*, New Jersey: Merck Sharpe & Dohme, 1981.

Fleming, A., ed. *Penicillin: Its Practical Application*. London: Butterworth, 1946.

Levy, S. B. *The Antibiotic Paradox*. New York: Plenum Press, 1992.

McFarlane, G. *Alexander Fleming: The Man and the Myth*. London: Chatto & Windus, 1984.

Chapter 2. The Effects of the Use and Abuse of Antibiotics

Barnes, P. F. and S. A. Barrows. "Tuberculosis in the 1990s." *Annals of Internal Medicine* 119(5) (1993): 400–410.

Cantekin, E.I., et al. "Anti-Microbial Therapy for Otitis Media With Effusion." *Journal of the American Medical Association* 266(23) (1991): 3309–3317.

Diamont, M. and B. Diamont. "Abuse and Timing of Antibiotics in Acute Otitis Media." *Archives of Otolaryngology* 100 (1974): 226–232.

Hauser, W. E. and J. S. Remington. "Effect of Antibiotics on the Immune System." *American Journal of Medicine* 72(5) (1982): 711–715.

Laurence, D. R and P. N. Bennett. *Clinical Pharmacology*. Edinburgh: Churchill Livingstone, 1980.

Londymore-Lim, L. *Poisonous Prescriptions*. Australia: Prevention of Disease & Disability, 1994.

Neu, H. C. and S. P. Henry. "Testing the Physician's Knowledge of Antibiotic Use." *New England Journal of Medicine* 293 (1975): 1291.

Chapter 3. Bacterial Resistance to Antibiotics

Barnes, P. F. and S. A. Barrows. "Tuberculosis in the 1990s." *Annals of Internal Medicine* 119(5) (1993): 400–410.

Bloom, B. R. and C. J. Murray. "Tuberculosis: Commentary on a Re-Emergent Killer." *Science* 257 (1992): 1055–1064.

Chandler, D. and A. E. Dugdale. "What Do Patients Know About Antibiotics?" *British Medical Journal* 8 (1976): 422.

Holmberg, S. O., et al. "Drug Resistant *Salmonella* From Animals Fed Anti-Microbials." *New England Journal of Medicine* 10 (1984): 311.

Kitamoto, O. et al. "On the Drug Resistance of *Shigella* Strains Isolated in 1955." *Journal of the Japanese Association for BactInfectious Diseases* 30 (1956): 403–405.

Kunin, C. M. "Resistance to Anti-Microbial Drugs—A Worldwide Calamity." *Annals of Internal Medicine* 118(7) (1993): 557–561.

Leclercq, R., et al. "Plasmid-Mediated Resistance to Vancomycin and Teicoplanin in *Enterococcus faecium.*" *New England Journal of Medicine* 319(3) (1988): 157–161.

Levy, S. B. "Antibiotic Availability and Use: Consequences to Man and His Environment." *Journal of Clinical Epidemiology* 44 Suppl. 2 (1991): 835–875.

_____. "Confronting Multi-Drug Resistance: A Role for Each of Us." *Journal of the American Medical Association* 269(14) (1993): 1840–1842.

Levy, S. B., J. Burke, and E. Wallace, eds. "Antibiotic Use and Antibiotic Resistance Worldwide." *Review of Infectious Diseases* 9 Suppl. 3 (1987): 5231–5316.

Mcleod, G. *A Veterinary Materia Medica.* Essex: Saffron Walden, 1983.

Mare, I. J. "Incidence of R-Factors Among Gram-Negative Bacteria in Drug-Free Human and Animal Communities." *Nature* 220 (1968) 1046–1047.

Mare, I. J. and J. N. Coetze. "The Incidence of Transmissible Drug Resistance Factors Among Strains of *E. coli* in the Pretoria Area." *South African Medical Journal* 40 (1966): 620–622.

Monaghan, C., et al. "Antibiotic Resistance and R-Factors in the Faecal Coliform Flora of Urban and Rural Dogs." *Antimicrobial Agents and Chemotherapy* (1981).

Ochiai, K., T. Totani, and Y. Toshiki. "*Shigella* Strains Resistant to Three Antibiotics. Epidemic Caused by Triply Resistant *Shigella* Strains in Nagoya." Nihon Iji Shimpo 1837 (1959): 25–37.

Ofek, I., et al. "Anti E. Coli Adhesion Activity of Cranberry and Blueberry Juices." *New England Journal of Medicine* 324(22) (1991): 1599.

Schwalbe, R. S., J. T. Stapleton, and P. H. Gilligan. "Emergence of

Vancomycin Resistance in Coagulase-Negative Staphylococci." *New England Journal of Medicine* 316(15) (1987) 927–931.

Skurray, R. A., et al. "Multi-Resistant *Staphylococcus Aureus*: Genetics and Evolution of Epidemic Australian Strains." *Journal of Antimicrobial Chemotherapy* Suppl. C (1988): 19–39.

Swartz, W., et al. *Human Health Risks With the Subtherapeutic Use of Penicillins* or *Tetracyclines in Animal Feed*. Washington, DC: National Academy Press, 1989.

Welch, G. H., "Antibiotic Resistance: A New Kind of Epidemic." *Postgraduate Medicine* 6 (1984): 76.

Wolfe, S. M. "Antibiotics." *Health Letter*. Washington, DC: The Public Citizens Health Research Group, 1989.

Chapter 4. The Treatment of Childhood Infections

Bain, J., E. Murphy, and F. Ross. "Acute Otitis Media: Clinical Cause Among Children Who Received a Short Course of High-Dose Antibiotic." *British Medical Journal* 291 (1985): 1243–1246.

Cantekin, E. I., et al. "Anti-Microbial Therapy for Otitis Media With Effusion." *Journal of the American Medical Association* 266(23) (1991): 3309–3317.

Freinberg, N. and T. Lyte. "Adjunctive Ascorbic Acid Administration and Antibiotic Therapy." *Journal of Dental Research* 36 (1957): 260–262.

Hull, D. and D. I. Johnston. *Essential Paediatrics*. Edinburgh: Churchill Livingstone, 1981.

Kendig, E. L. *Disorders of the Respiratory Tract in Children*. Philadelphia: Saunders, 1977.

Klein, J. O. "Microbiology and Management of Otitis Media." *Paediatrician* 8 Suppl. 1 (1979): 10–25.

Krugman, S., R. Ward, and S. L. Katz. *Infectious Diseases of Children*. St Louis: Mosby, 1977.

Schmidt, M. A. *Childhood Ear Infections: What Every Parent and Physician Should Know.* California: North Atlantic Books, 1990.

Williams, H. E. and P. D. Phelan. *Respiratory Illness in Children.* Oxford: Blackwell Scientific, 1975.

Chapter 5. Herbal Medicine

Beuscher, N. and L. Kopanski. "Stimulation of the Immune Response With Substances Derived From *Baptisia Tinctoria.*" *Planta Medica 5* (1985): 381–384.

Beuscher, N., H. Beuscher, and C. Bodinet. *Enhanced Release of Interleukin-I From Mouse Macrophages by Glycoproteins and Polysaccharides From Baptisia Tinctoria and Echinacea spp.* Braunschweig, Germany: 37th Annual Congress on Medicinal Plant Research, 1989.

British Herbal Medicine Association Scientific Committee. *British Herbal Pharmacopoeia,* Vols. 1, 2 & 3, London: British Herbal Medicine Association, 1983.

Coeugneit, E. and R. Kühnast. "Recurrent Candidiasis Adjuvant Immuno-Therapy With Different Formulations of Echinacea." *Therapiewoche* 36 (1986): 3352.

Culbreth, D. *A Manual of Materia Medica and Pharmacology.* Oregon: Ecletic Medical Publications, 1983.

Freyer, H. U. "Frequency of Common Infections in Childhood and Likelihood of Prophylaxis." *Fortschritte der Therapie* 92 (1974): 165.

Goullon, H. *Thuja Occidentalis,* Leipzig, Germany: Gustav Engelverlag.

Grieve, M. *A Modern Herbal.* New York: Dover, 1971.

Halter, K. "Innerliche Behandlung juveniler Warzen mit Thuja occidentalis." *Dermatologische Wochenschrift* 120 (1949): 353–55.

Hobbs, C. *The Echinacea Handbook*. California: Botanica Press, 1989.

James, J. *AIDS Treatment News* 19 (1986).

Khurana, S. M. P. "Effect of Homeopathic Drugs on Plant Viruses." *Planta Medica* 20 (1971): 142–146.

Lloyd, J. U. *A Treatise on Echinacea*. Cincinnati: Lloyd Brothers, 1917.

McLoughlin, G. "Echinacea: A Literature Review," *Australian Journal of Medical Herbalism* 4 (1992): 104—111.

Moerman, D. E. *American Medical Ethno-Botany*. New York: Garland Publishers, 1977.

Mowrey, D. B. *The Scientific Validation of Herbal Medicine*. New Canaan, Connecticut: Keats Publishing, 1986.

Smith, Ed. *The Therapeutic Herb Manual*. 1993.

Wacker, A. and W. Hilbig. "Virus Inhibition by Echinacea Purpurea." *Planta Medica* 33 (1978): 89.

Weiss, R. F. *Lehrbuch der Phytotherapie*. Stuttgart, Germany: Hippocrates Verlag, 1980.

Wren, R. C. and R. W. Wren, eds. *Potter's New Cyclopaedia of Botanical Drugs* and *Preparations*. Holsworthy Health Science Press, 1975.

Chapter 6. Homeopathic Medicine

Campbell, A. *The Two Faces of Homeopathy*. London: Hale, 1984.

Castro, D. and G. Nogueira. "Use of the Nosode Meningococcinum as a Preventive Against Meningitis." *Journal of the American Institute of Homeopathy* 68 (1975): 211—219.

Castro, M. *The Complete Homeopathy Handbook*. London: Macmillan, 1990.

Coulter, H. L. *Homeopathic Science and Modern Medicine*: The *Physics of Healing with Microdoses*. Berkeley, California: North Atlantic Books, 1987.

Gaucher, C., D. Jeulin, and P. Peycru. "Homeopathic Treatment of Cholera in Peru: An Initial Clinical Study." *British Homeopathic Journal* 81 (1992): 18–21.

Reckweg, H. H. *Materia Medica Homeopathica Anti-Homotoxica*. Baden-Baden, Germany: Aurelia Verlag, 1983.

Schmidt, M. A., L. H. Smith, and K. W. Sehnert. *Beyond Antibiotics*. Berkeley, California: North Atlantic Books, 1993.

Tyler, M. *Homeopathic Drug Pictures*. London: Health Science Press, 1970.

Vithoulkas, G. *Homeopathy: Medicine of the New Man*. Wellingborough: Thorsons, 1985.

_____. *The Science of Homeopathy*. Wellingborough: Thorsons, 1986.

Chapter 7. Nutritional Supplementation

Al-Nakib, M., et al. "Prophylaxis and Treatment of Rhinovirus Colds with Zinc Gluconate Lozenges." *Journal of Antimicrobial Chemotherapy* 20 (1987): 893–901.

Anderson, R., et al. "The Effects of Increasing Weekly Doses of Ascorbate on Certain Cellular and Hormonal Immune Functions in Normal Volunteers." *American Journal of Clinical Nutrition* 33 (1980): 71.

Beisel, W., et al. "Single Nutrient Effects of Immunologic Function." *Journal of the American Medical Association* 245 (1981): 53–58.

Bogden, J. D., et al. "Zinc and Immunocompetence in the Elderly: Baseline Data on Zinc and Immunity in Unsupplemental Subjects." *American Journal of Clinical Nutrition* 46 (1987): 101–109.

Bright-See, E. "Vitamin C and Cancer Prevention." *Seminars in Oncology* 10(3) (1983): 294–298.

Brody, I. "Topical Treatment of Recurrent Herpes Simplex and Post-Herpetic Erythema Multiforme With Low Concentrations of Zinc Sulphate Solution." *British Journal of Dermatology* 104 (1981): 191–194.

Bulkena, E. G. "Zinc Compounds, a New Treatment in Peptic Ulcer." *Drugs Under Experimental and Clinical Research* 15(2) (1989): 83–89.

Cameron, E. and L. Pauling. "Supplemental Ascorbate in the Supportive Treatment of Cancer: Prolongation of Survival Times in Terminal Human Cancer." *Proceedings of the National Academy of Sciences* 73 (1976): 3685.

Chandra, R. K. "Excessive Intake of Zinc Impairs Immune Responses." *Journal of the American Medical Association* 252 (1984): 1443–1446.

Cheraskin, E., W. M. Ringsdorf, and E. L. Sisley. *The Vitamin C Connection*. Wellingborough, Thorsons, 1983.

Dahl, H. and M. Degre. "The Effect of Ascorbic Acid on the Production of Human Interferon and the Anti-Viral Activity *in vitro*." *Acta Pathologica, Microbiologica et Immunologica Scandinavia* B 84 (1976): 280.

Dieter, M. "Further Studies on the Relationship Between Vitamin C and Thymic Hormonal Factor." *Proceedings of the Society for Experimental Biology and Medicine* 136 (1971): 316–322.

Duchateau, J., et al. "Beneficial Effects of Oral Zinc Supplementation on the Immune Response of Old People." *American Journal of Medicine* 70 (1981): 1001–1004.

Eby, G. A., D. A. Davis, and W. W. Halcomb. "Reduction in Duration of Common Colds by Zinc Gluconate Lozenges in a Double-Blind Study." *Antimicrobial Agents and Chemotherapy* 25 (1984): 20.

Fabris, N., et al. "AIDS, Zinc Deficiency and Thymic Hormone Failure." *Journal of the American Medical Association* 259 (1988): 839–840.

Fraser, R. C., et al. "The Effect of Variations in Vitamin C Intake on the Cellular Response of Guinea Pigs." *American Journal of Clinical Nutrition* 33 (1980): 839.

Frei, B., L. England. and B. N. Ames. "Ascorbate as an Outstanding Antioxidant in Human Blood Plasma." *Proceedings of the National Academy of Sciences* 86 (1989): 6377.

Hansen, M. A., G. Fernandes, and R. A. Good. "Nutrition and Immunity: The Influence of Diet on Auto-Immunity and the Role of Zinc in the Immune Response." *Annual Review of Nutrition* 2 (1982):151–177.

Hoffer, A. "Ascorbic Acid and Kidney Stones." *Canadian Medical Association Journal* 132 (1985): 320.

Hornig, D. *Vitamins and Minerals in Pregnancy and Lactation: Nestlé Nutrition Workshop Series*, No. 16, 433–4, New York: Raven Press, 1988.

Kalokerinos, A. *Every Second Child*. New Canaan, Connecticut: Keats Publishing, 1981.

Karlowski, T. R., et al. "Ascorbic Acid for the Common Cold: A Prophylactic and Therapeutic Trial." *Journal of the American Medical Association* 231 (1975): 1038.

Katz, E. and E. Margolith. "Inhibition of Vaccinia Virus Maturation by Zinc Chloride." *Antimicrobial Agents and Chemotherapy* 19 (1981): 213–217.

Kaul, T. N., E. Middleton, and P. Orga. "Antiviral Effect of Flavonoids on Human Viruses." *Journal of Medical Virology* 15 (1985): 71—79.

Klein, M. A. "The National Cancer Institute and Ascorbic Acid." *Townsend Letter for Doctors* (1991).

Klenner, F. R. "Virus Pneumonia and Its Treatment With Vitamin C." *Journal of Southern Medicine and Surgery* 2 (1948).

_____. "Massive Doses of Vitamin C and the Virus Diseases." *Journal of Southern Medicine and Surgery* 113(4) (1951).

_____. 'The Use of Vitamin C as an Antibiotic." *Journal of Applied Nutrition* 6 (1953).

Leibovitz, B. and B. V. Siegel. "Ascorbic Acid, Neutrophil Function and the Immune System." *International Journal of Vitamin and Nutrition Research* 48 (1978): 159.

Pauling, L. "Evolution and the Need for Ascorbic Acid." *Proceedings of the National Academy of Sciences* 67 (1970): 1643.

_____. "The Significance of the Evidence About Ascorbic Acid and the Common Cold." *Proceedings of the National Academy of Sciences* 68 (1971): 2678–2681.

_____. *How to Live Longer and Feel Better*. New York: W. H. Freeman, 1986.

_____. *Vitamin C and the Common Cold*. San Francisco: W. H. Freeman, 1970.

Prasar, A. "Clinical Biochemical and Nutritional Spectrum of Zinc Deficiency in Human Subjects: An Update." *Nutrition Review* 41 (1983): 197–208.

Rivers, J. M. "Safety of High Level Vitamin C Ingestion." Applied Nutrition 3rd Conference on Vitamin C, *Annals of the New York Academy of Science* 498 (1987): 445–454.

Romney, S. L., et al. "Plasma Vitamin C and Uterine Cervical Dysplasia." *American Journal of Obstetrics and Gynecology* 151 (1985): 976–980.

Scott, J. "On the Biochemical Similarities of Ascorbic Acid and Interferon." *Journal of Theoretical Biology* 98 (1982): 235–238.

Shilotri, P. G. and K. S. Bhat. "Effect of Megadoses of Vitamin C on Bactericidal Activity of Leukocytes." *American Journal of Clinical Nutrition* 30 (1977): 1077.

Siegel, B. V. "Enhanced Interferon Response to Murine Leukaemia Virus by Ascorbic Acid." *Infection and Immunity* 10 (1974): 409.

Siegel, B. V. and J. I. Morton. "Vitamin C and Immunity: Influence of Ascorbate on PGE2 Synthesis and Implications for Natural Killer Cell Activity." *International Journal of Vitamin and Nutrition Research* 54 (1984): 339.

Stone, I. *The Healing Factor: Vitamin C Against Disease*. New York: Gromet & Dunlop, 1972.

Chapter 8. Bacterial Supplementation

Alm, I., et al. "The Regulatory and Protective Role of the Normal Microflora." *Wenner-Gren International Symposium Series* (1988).

Barefoot, S. and T. R. Klaenhammer. "Detection and Activity of Lactacin B, a Bacteriocin Produced by *Lactobacillus acidophilus.*" *Applied and Environmental Microbiology* 45 (1983): 1808.

Bullen, C. L., P. V. Tearle, and A. T. Willis. "Bifidobacteria in the Intestinal Tract of Infants: An *in vivo* Study." *Journal of Medical Microbiology* 9 (1975): 325.

Byssen, H. "Role of the Gut Micro-Flora in Metabolism of Lipids and Sterols." *Proceedings of the Nutrition Society* 32 (1973): 59.

Colombel, J. F., et al. "Yoghurt with Bifidobacterium Longum Reduces Erythromycin-Induced Gastro-Intestinal Effects." *The Lancet* 2 (1987): 43.

Goldin, B. R. and S. L. Gorbach. "Alterations of the Intestinal Flora by Diet, Oral Antibiotics and Lactobacillus." *Journal of the National Cancer Institute* 73 (1984): 689.

Gordon, D., J. Macrea, and D. M. Wheater. "A Lactobacillus Preparation for Use With Antibiotics." *The Lancet* 272 (1957): 889.

Hamdan, I. T., et al. "Acidolin: An Antibiotic Produced by Lactobacillus Acidophilus." *Journal of Antibiotics* 27 (1974): 631.

Kim, H. S. and S. E. Gilliland. "Lactobacillus Acidophilus as a Dietary Adjunct for Milk to Aid Lactose Digestion in Humans." *Journal of Dairy Science* 66 (1983): 959.

Lipid Research Clinics Program. "The Lipid Research Clinics Coronary Primary Prevention Trials Results: Reduction in the Incidence of Coronary Heart Disease." *Journal of the American Medical Association* 251 (1984): 351

Mann, G. V. "A Factor in Yoghurt Which Lowers Cholesteremia in Man." *Atherosclerosis* 26(3) (1977): 335—340.

Mann, G. V. and A. Spoerry. "Studies of a Surfactant and Cholesteremia in the Masai." *American Journal of Clinical Nutrition* 27 (1974): 464.

Shahani, K. M. and A. Ayebo. "Role of Dietary Lactobacilli in the Gastro-Intestinal Microecology." *American Journal of Clinical Nutrition* 33 (1980): 2448.

Vogel, H. C. A. *The Nature Doctor*. Edinburgh, Scotland: Mainstream, 1990.

Chapter 9. A Healthy Diet: A Form of Nutritional Medicine

Beukes, V. *Killer Foods of the Twentieth Century*. Johannesburg, South Africa: Perskor, 1974.

Bieler, H. M. *Food is Your Best Medicine*. London: Neville Spearman, 1968.

Budd, M. L. *Low Blood Sugar (Hypoglycaemia)—The 20th Century Epidemic?* Wellingborough: Thorsons, 1984.

Chavance, M., et al. "Nutritional Support Improves Antibody Response to Influenza Virus in the Elderly." *British Medical Journal* 11(9) (1985): 1348–1349.

Cheraskin, E. *Diet and Disease*, New Canaan, Connecticut: Keats Publishing, 1968.

Dietary Goals for the United States. Washington DC: U.S. Senate Select Committee on Nutrition and Human Needs, 1977.

Jensen, Bernard and Mark Andersen. *Empty Harvest*. Garden City Park, NY: Avery Publishing Group, 1990.

Kumar, A., M. Weatherly, and D. C. Beaman. "Sweeteners, Flavourings and Dyes in Antibiotic Preparations." *Paediatrics* 87(3) (1991): 352–359.

Millstone, E. and J. Abraham. *Additives*. London: Penguin, 1988.

Newberne, P. and G. Williams. "Nutritional Influences on the Course of Infections." In *Resistance to Infectious Disease*, ed Dunlop, R. H. and H. W. Moon, Canada: Saskatoon Modern Press, 1970.

Pfeiffer, C. C. *Total Nutrition*. London: Granada, 1982.

Sanchez, A., et al. "Role of Sugar in Human Neutrophilic Phagocytosis." *American Journal of Clinical Nutrition* 26 (1973): 180.

Sandler, B. P. *Diet Prevents Polio*. The Lee Foundation for Nutritional Research, 1951.

Stitt, P. A. *Fighting the Food Giants*. Wisconsin: Natural Press, 1980.

Ward, N. I., et al. "The Influence of the Chemical Additive Tartrazine on the Zinc Status of Hyperactive Children—A Double-Blind Placebo-Controlled Study." *Journal of Nutritional Medicine* 1 (1990): 51–57.

Williams, R. J. *Nutrition Against Disease*. London: Pitman, 1971.

Wilson, F. A. *Food Fit for Humans*. London: Daniel, 1975.

Chapter 10. Stress and the Immune System

Angier, N. "Chronic Anger is a Major Health Risk: Studies Find." *New York Times* (December 13 1990) (from papers presented at the 1990 conference of the American Heart Association).

Benson, H. *The Relaxation Response*. New York: Morrow, 1975.

Bombardelli, E., A. Cirstoni, and A. Liehi. "The Effect of Acute and Chronic Ginseng Saponins Treatment on Adrenal Function." Proceedings of the 3rd International Ginseng Symposium, 1980.

Boyce, T. W., et al. "Influence of Life Events and Family Routines on Childhood Respiratory Tract Illness." *Paediatrics* 60(4) (1977): 609–615.

Cohen, S., D. Tyrrell, and A. Smith. "Psychological Stress and Susceptibility to the Common Cold." *New England Journal of Medicine* 325 (1991): 606–612.

D'Angelo, L., et al. "A Double-Blind Placebo Controlled Clinical Study on the Effect of a Standardised Ginseng Extract on Psychomotor Performance in Healthy Volunteers." *Journal of Ethnopharmacology* 16 (1986): 15–22.

Fulder, S. J. "Ginseng and the Hypothalamic-Pituitary Control of Stress." *American Journal of Chinese Medicine* 9 (1981): 112–118.

Hoffman, D. *The New Holistic Herbal*. London: Element, 1990.

Holmes, T. H. and R. H. Rahe. "The Social Readjustment Scale." *Journal of Psychosomatic Research* 11, (1967): 213–218 [Reproduced with permission].

Moldofsky, H., et al. "The Relationship of Interleukin-I and Immune Functions to Sleep in Humans." *Psychosomatic Medicine* 48 (1986): 309–315.

Pizzorno, J. E. and M. T. Murray. *A Textbook of Natural Medicine*. Rocklin, California: Prima, 1988.

Seyle, H. *Stress in Health and Disease*. London: Butterworths, 1976.

Simonton, O. C., S. Matthews-Simonton, and J. L. Creighton. *Getting Well Again*. London: Bantam, 1980.

Sobel, D. and R. Ornstein. *Healthy Pleasures*. Reading, Massachusetts: Addison-Wesley, 1989.

INDEX